Mable Hoffman's

CHOCOLATE COOKERY

Contents

ANOTHER BEST-SELLING COOKERY VOLUME FROM H.P.BOOKS

Authors: Mable & Gar Hoffman; Publisher: Helen Fisher; Editor: Carlene Tejada; Senior Editor: Jon Latimer; Editor-in-Chief: Carl Shipman; Art Director: Don Burton; Book Design & Assembly: Laura Hardock, Tom Jakeway; Typography: Connie Brown, Cindy Coatsworth, Judy Smith, Kris Spitler; Research Assistants: Jan Robertson, Linda Worsham; Food Stylist: Mable Hoffman; Photography: George deGennaro Studios—George deGennaro, David Wong, Dennis Skinner, Tom Miyasaki.

Published by H.P.Books, P.O. Box 5367, Tucson, AZ 85703 602/888-2150

ISBN: Softcover, 0-89586-016-3; Hardcover, 0-89586-017-1
Library of Congress Catalog Card Number, 78-61007
© 1978 Fisher Publishing, Inc.
Printed in U.S.A.

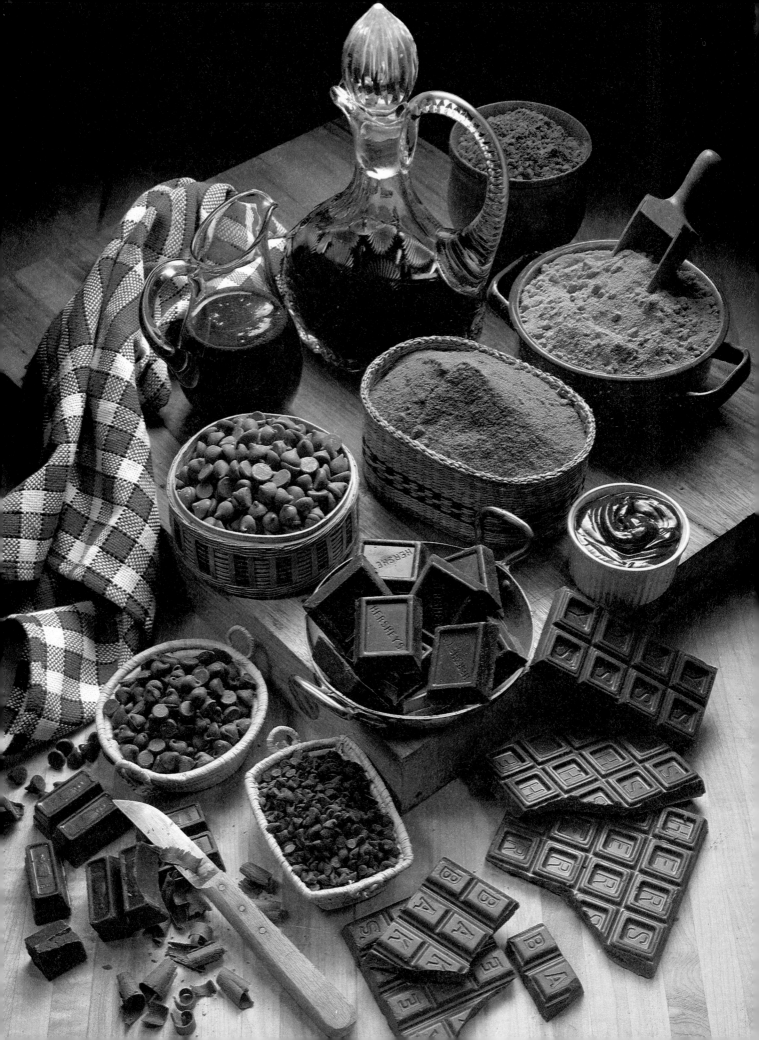

The World's Favorite Flavor

No other flavor has ever rivaled chocolate in universal appeal. Since days of Montezuma when the Aztecs drank it from golden goblets in elaborate ceremonies, chocolate has been held in high esteem. The cocoa beans that Cortez brought back to Spain were so highly prized they were kept secret from the rest of Europe for nearly a century. Eventually its popularity spread and drinking chocolate, the only way it was served, became very fashionable. *Chocolate houses,* cafes serving chocolate drinks, sprang up in England and Holland. It wasn't until the 19th Century that the Swiss developed a method of making solid milk chocolate.

The enchantment of chocolate has grown through the years. Thanks to the ingenuity of today's chocolate manufacturers, the selection of chocolate products is almost mind-boggling. This book describes the principal products to make it easier for you to choose which to use for a particular recipe. We have tried to give you a representative group of recipes using each of these chocolate products. These recipes have been carefully tested with the kind of chocolate indicated in each. If you try the recipe with another chocolate, you will probably get slightly different results. If you find it necessary to substitute one chocolate for another, please use the amounts suggested in our Table of Substitutions on page 5.

Main Types Of Chocolate Products

Unsweetened Chocolate Squares do not contain sugar or flavorings. The 8-ounce package contains 8 individually wrapped 1-ounce squares which are grooved to break easily into 1/2-ounce pieces. Sometimes it is called *unsweetened baking chocolate.* Older recipes may refer to it as *bitter chocolate.*

Semisweet Chocolate Squares contain unsweetened chocolate blended with sugar, cocoa butter and flavorings. The 8-ounce package contains 8 individually wrapped 1-ounce squares which are grooved to break into 1/2-ounce pieces. Older recipes may call them *dot chocolate.*

Semisweet Chocolate Pieces contain unsweetened chocolate blended with sugar, cocoa butter and flavorings. They are available in 6- and 12-ounce bags. Small teardrop-shaped pieces are about 2/5 inch across the base and about 2/5 inch tall. The exact name varies according to the manufacturer. They may be referred to as chocolate bits, morsels or chips. The 6-ounce bag contains 1 cup of pieces; the 12-ounce bag measures 2 cups.

Sweet Cooking Chocolate is a special blend of chocolate with sugar and cocoa butter. It is available in a 4-ounce bar which is grooved into 18 sections so you can use part of the bar. Its most popular use has been in making German Chocolate Cake. Do not confuse the sweet cooking chocolate bar with a regular milk chocolate candy bar.

Dark Chocolate Flavor Baking Chips is cocoa blended with sugar, vegetable oil and flavorings. Small and minature dark pieces are available in 6- and 12-ounce bags. During baking, these pieces soften slightly but hold their shape. They are not as readily available as semisweet chocolate pieces.

Milk Chocolate is chocolate liquor combined with extra cocoa butter, milk or cream, sugar and flavorings. The best known product is the popular milk chocolate candy bar which is available in .5 ounce, 1.05 ounces, 4 ounces and 8 ounces. It is also available in foil-wrapped kisses and novelty shapes such as Christmas bells or Easter eggs. The milk chocolate pieces, which are the same size and shape as semisweet chocolate pieces, are ideal for cooking. The are available in most markets in bags weighing about 6 ounces or 12 ounces.

Pre-Melted Unsweetened Baking Chocolate is a blend of cocoa and vegetable oil that has been pre-melted. It is available in cartons containing 8 1-ounce packets that you tear open and then squeeze out the chocolate. It is labled "unsweetened chocolate flavor for baking" and is semi-liquid so you can use it without melting or measuring.

Chocolate Sprinkles are tiny cylindrical chocolate decorations usually found on grocery shelves near cake decorating supplies. They are handy for dipping small candies or cookies or for sprinkling over tops of cakes, pies or ice cream.

Unsweetened Cocoa is unsweetened cocoa powder with varying amounts of cocoa butter. Regular cocoa contains about 16 per cent cocoa butter. *Dutch Process Cocoa*, with stronger flavor and color, has been specially treated. When using unsweetened cocoa in our recipe ingredient lists we use the term "unsweetened cocoa powder" so you will know to use unsweetened powder right from the container rather than a mix or blend.

Hot Cocoa Mix contains cocoa, sugar and milk solids. It is designed especially to make a fast beverage by adding hot water. It comes in several different sized boxes with individual 1-ounce envelopes as well as in bulk in 1- or 2-pound cans.

Powdered Chocolate Flavoring for Milk is a blend of cocoa, sugar and flavorings which dissolves easily in hot or cold milk. Brand names such as Hershey's Instant and Nestlé Quik are usually available in 1- or 2-pound cans. It is handy for cooking when a sweet milk chocolate is desired.

Chocolate Flavored Syrup is a mixture of cocoa, sugar, corn syrup and flavorings. It is available in 5-1/2-ounce and 1-pound cans. It is very popular as a sauce, topping or in beverages.

Chocolate Fudge Topping is a blend of cocoa, sugar, corn syrup and flavorings with milk, cream or butter. Like chocolate syrup but thicker, it is usually available in a 1-pound can or jar.

Chocolate Liqueurs come in a variety of flavors. *Crème de cacao,* both the chocolate color and transparent variety, is one of the most popular. The transparent or white crème de cacao is used in recipes where chocolate color is not desired. You can also find mint, coconut, cherry and orange-flavored chocolate liqueurs.

Chocolate Cookies used for the pie crusts and cheesecake crusts in this book are two types. The *chocolate snap*, similar in size and shape to the ginger snap, is easy to crush and combines well with other ingredients. The *chocolate wafer* is flat, thin and dark chocolate color. It can be used whenever the chocolate snap is used but is harder to handle.

Substituting Chocolate Products

The recipes in this book were tested with the specific chocolate listed in each recipe. If you do not have the product listed, here are a few suggested substitutes.

● Substitute equal amounts of pre-melted unsweetened baking chocolate for unsweetened chocolate, and vice versa.

● Substitute 3 tablespoons unsweetened cocoa plus 1 tablespoon shortening for 1 ounce unsweetened chocolate.

● Substitute 2 ounces unsweetened chocolate, 7 tablespoons sugar and 2 tablespoons shortening for each cup or 6 ounces of semisweet chocolate pieces.

● Semisweet chocolate pieces and semisweet chocolate squares can be melted and used interchangeably. If not melted, chocolate pieces retain their shape and soften only slightly when baked. Semisweet chocolate squares must be melted, cut up or grated before being added to other ingredients.

How To Melt Chocolate

Melting chocolate is not as simple as putting chocolate in a saucepan and placing it on the stove until you're ready for it. *Never* leave chocolate on the heat unless you are close by. Chocolate scorches easily and once scorched, cannot be used.

There are four ways to melt chocolate successfully. Choose the one that's best for you and proceed with care.

Over hot water—Place chocolate in the top of a double boiler. Place top of double boiler over hot but *not* boiling water until chocolate is almost melted. Remove top of double boiler from hot water; stir chocolate until smooth. For small amounts, place chocolate in a custard cup or small bowl. Set cup or bowl in a pan of hot but not boiling water until chocolate is almost melted.

Remove cup or bowl from water; stir chocolate until smooth.

In a microwave oven—Place chocolate in a custard cup or glass measuring cup. Heat in microwave oven for 1 or 2 minutes. The time varies with the amount of chocolate.

Over direct heat—This must be handled very carefully. Melt chocolate in a small heavy saucepan or skillet over very low heat, stirring constantly. Remove from heat as soon as chocolate melts. Or, set saucepan with chocolate over the pilot light; stir occasionally until melted.

In the oven—Place a small ovenproof bowl with chocolate in the oven after the oven has been turned off and is no longer hot but still warm. Check the chocolate frequently to be sure it's not burning.

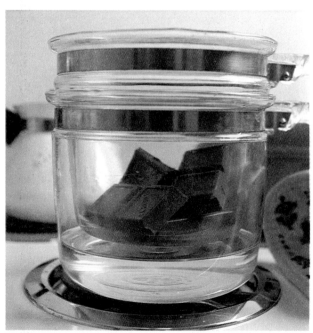

Chocolate can be melted over hot water.

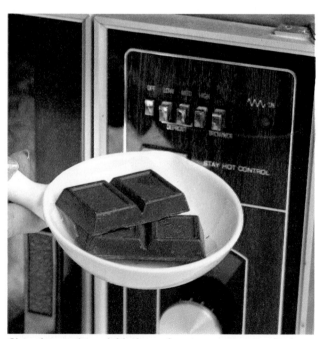

Chocolate melts quickly in a microwave oven.

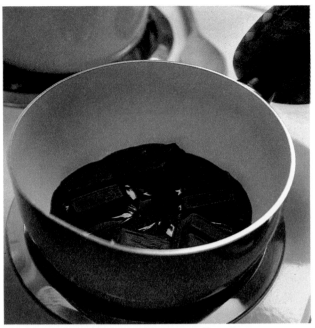
Use extra care to melt chocolate over direct heat.

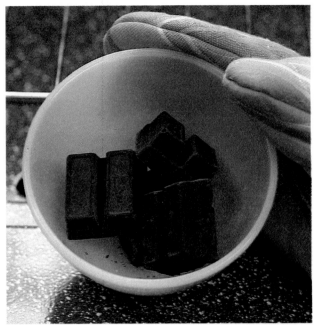
To melt chocolate in your oven, be sure the oven is off.

TIPS FOR MELTING CHOCOLATE

• Unsweetened chocolate has a tendency to liquefy when melted, but semisweet, sweet cooking and milk chocolate will hold their shapes when melted until stirred.

• Squares of chocolate melt easier and faster when cut into chunks or small pieces.

• *Never* add water to melting chocolate unless specified in the recipe. Water will not make chocolate more liquid. Instead it will cause chocolate to stiffen and prevent it from being smooth. If melted chocolate is too thick, thin it with a small amount of vegetable shortening.

• Don't try to hurry the melting process by turning up the heat. High temperatures will thicken or scorch the chocolate.

• Chocolate will continue to melt after it is removed from heat, so you can partly melt it, remove it from heat, then stir until smooth.

Handle With Care

STORAGE

Store chocolate products in a cool place, preferably below 75°F (25°C), but not in the refrigerator. When chocolate is kept at higher temperatures, the cocoa butter begins to melt and the surface of the chocolate becomes gray. This is known as *bloom.* It doesn't affect the flavor but it has an unappetizing appearance. Keep chocolate in a dry place. Any moisture that seeps inside the package is likely to change the chocolate's texture.

COOKING

Chocolate, even when combined with other ingredients, scorches easily. Use low or moderate heat when cooking a chocolate mixture on top of the stove. It is a good idea to stir the mixture while it is cooking to keep it well mixed and to avoid scorching. When making candy, do not stir chocolate mixtures that are cooking unless instructed to do so by the recipe.

Decorating With Chocolate

Grated Chocolate is an easy and fast way to dress up a pie, custard or cake. Most graters have two grating sections, one finer than the other. Use the size most flattering to the dish you are decorating.

Even if you only need to grate a small amount of chocolate, a large, thick piece is easier to grate than a small, thin piece. For easy clean-up, hold the grater on aluminum foil or wax paper. With the grater at an angle, rub the chocolate across it.

To grate larger amounts, hold the chocolate with a paper towel so the heat of your hand doesn't melt it. A *mouli* grater is faster and more convenient than hand grating, and the chocolate is grated uniformly. You can grate chocolate in a blender if you cut it into small chunks first. However, the pieces will not be uniform in size and the friction of the blades is likely to melt the chocolate.

Chocolate Leaves are easy to make. Wash an assortment of leaves from non-poisonous plants such as roses or geraniums. Pat dry with paper towels. Melt semisweet chocolate squares or a combination of milk chocolate pieces mixed with semisweet chocolate. With a narrow spatula or knife, spread a layer of melted chocolate about 1/8 inch thick on the *back* of each leaf just to the edge. Try not to let any chocolate spill over to the front side of leaf. Place on flat pan or tray. Chill until firm. Carefully peel off leaves. Use leaf-shaped chocolate to decorate cakes or other desserts.

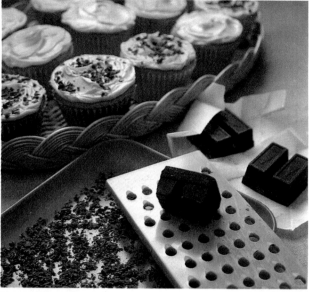

Grated Chocolate

Drizzled Chocolate or Allegretti Decoration is another easy way to dress up a layer cake or an angel-food cake. First, frost the cake with your favorite white frosting. Swirl the sides and the top with a spatula. Let the cake stand until the frosting is firm. Melt 1 square of semisweet chocolate with 1/2 teaspoon of shortening. Cool slightly. Drizzle the melted mixture from the tip of a teaspoon around the top edge of the frosted cake. Some of the chocolate will drip down the sides of the cake.

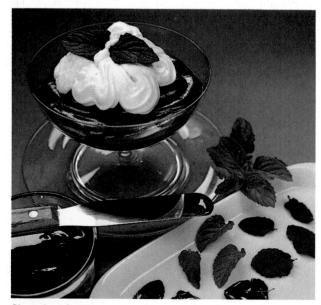

Chocolate Leaves

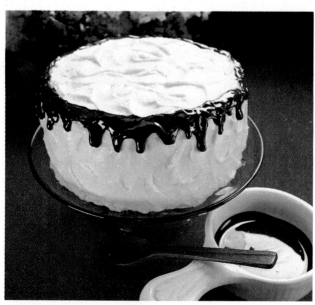

Drizzled Chocolate or Allegretti Decoration

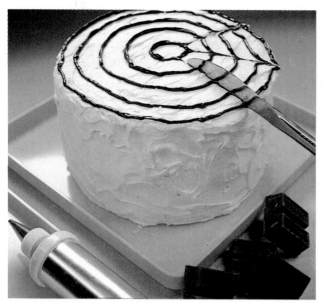

Chocolate Spiderweb Design

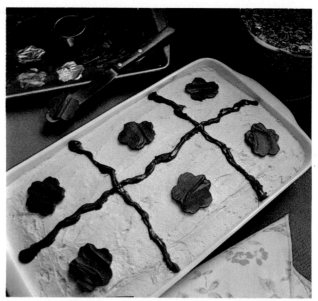

Decorative Chocolate Cut-Outs

A **Chocolate Spiderweb Design** is an unusual but easy-to-make decoration for the top of a cake. First frost a 2- or 3-layer cake with your favorite white frosting. Let the cake stand until the frosting is firm. Melt semisweet chocolate and let it stand until it is almost cool but not set. Spoon the cooled melted chocolate into a pastry tube or cake decorator. Attach a tip with 1 small plain hole. Pipe the chocolate through the pastry tube, making 5 or 6 circles around the top of the cake. Immediately pull the dull edge of a table knife across the chocolate circles from the center to the outer edge. Do this 8 to 10 times across the top of the cake.

Chocolate Curls are not difficult but the temperature of the chocolate is important. It should be slightly warm so the curls will not crack, but not warm enough to melt. Unwrap the chocolate. Place it on foil or wax paper. Let unsweetened and semisweet squares stand 15 to 20 minutes at about 90°F (30°C). Milk chocolate should stand at a slightly lower temperature. Use a gas oven with a pilot light or an electric oven that has been warmed slightly then turned off. Thinly shave the chocolate with a swivel-bladed vegetable peeler. Long strokes, with the peeler going diagonally across the smooth side of chocolate, produce larger and longer curls. Carefully insert a toothpick or small skewer into the curl to pick it up and place it on the dessert.

Decorative Chocolate Cut-Outs make effective seasonal designs. Line a cookie sheet with aluminum foil. Melt semisweet chocolate pieces; pour onto the foil-lined cookie sheet. Cool until almost set. Cut into desired designs. Use cookie cutters for large decorations, canapé cutters for small designs, or outline your own with the point of a sharp knife. Do not remove cut-outs from pan. Return pan to cool place until chocolate is firm. Insert spatula under each cut-out and remove from pan. Use as decorations for pies or cakes.

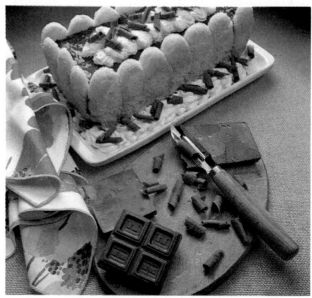

Chocolate Curls

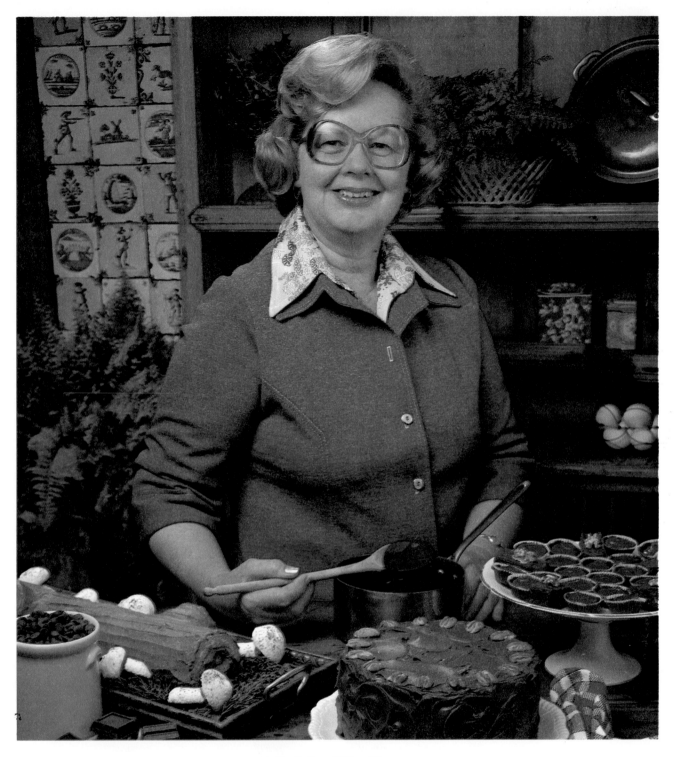

Mable Hoffman

Mable Hoffman loves to cook and has been doing it professionally for most of her life. Even before her first book, *Crockery Cookery,* zoomed to the top of the bestseller lists in 1975, Mable was an accomplished and sought-after food stylist and consultant. Mable's *Crepe Cookery,* issued in 1976, was a repeat bestseller. Both books won the R. T. French Tastemaker Award, the "Oscar" for cook-

books, as the best softcover cookbooks of the year. Mable's third book, *Mini Deep-Fry Cookery,* continued her series of winning books.

But *Chocolate Cookery* is something even more special; a labor of love. For years Mable has been collecting the world's favorite chocolate recipes and now she shares the best and most delicious with you!

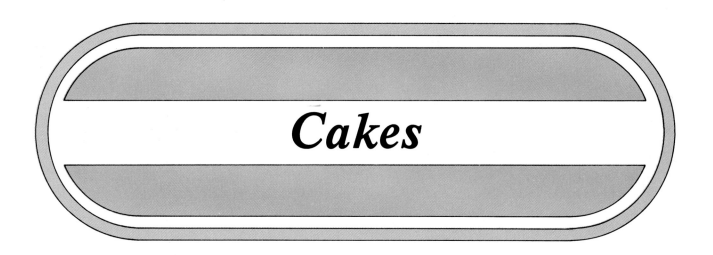

Cakes

Cakes have always been associated with celebrations and special occasions. We bake heart-shaped cakes for Valentines, honor Mother on her day with a cake, pack a cake for the 4th of July picnic, and bake a variety of cakes for the holidays. And who wants to celebrate a birthday without a cake!

To help you with all your special celebrations, or to make any day special, we have assembled an unbelievable collection of chocolate cakes. We've included cherished recipes handed down from one generation to another and in many cases we have developed streamlined versions of these classics.

Here are some hints to help you bake the perfect cake: First, assemble all the ingredients before you begin mixing. Butter or margarine will cream easier if brought to room temperature. In an effort to save time, effort and dishwashing, we have avoided the extra step of sifting flour wherever possible. There are a few exceptions with cake flour when

the cakes are very delicate in texture. To measure flour, use a spoon to scoop it out of the bag or canister. Never pack flour in the measuring cup. To make a level measurement, pull the dull edge of a straight knife across the top of the cup. If the dry ingredients are combined before being mixed into the batter, you can cut down on dishwashing by using a sheet of foil or wax paper instead of an additional bowl.

Instead of repeating the various ways to tell when a cake is done in each recipe, we suggest you try one or more of the following tests. Your cake is done:
- If it has pulled away from the sides of the pan.
- If you lightly touch the center of the cake and the top springs back leaving no imprint of your finger.
- If a toothpick or cake tester inserted into the center of the cake comes out clean.

Best Fudge Cake

Our very best chocolate cake made with unsweetened chocolate—a 2-layer delight!

3 oz. unsweetened chocolate
1/2 cup butter or margarine
2-1/4 cups light brown sugar, lightly packed
3 eggs
1-1/2 teaspoons vanilla extract

2 teaspoons baking soda
1/2 teaspoon salt
2-1/4 cups sifted cake flour
1 cup dairy sour cream
1 cup boiling water

Melt chocolate; set aside. Grease and flour two 9-inch cake pans; set aside. Preheat oven to 350°F (175°C). In a large mixer bowl, cream butter or margarine until smooth. Add brown sugar and eggs. Beat with electric mixer on high speed until light and fluffy, about 5 minutes. With mixer on low speed, beat in vanilla and melted chocolate, then baking soda and salt. Add flour alternately with sour cream, beating on low speed until smooth. Pour in boiling water; stir with a spoon until blended. Pour into prepared pans. Bake 35 minutes or until done. Cool in pans 10 minutes. Turn out on wire racks. Cool completely. Frost, if desired. Makes one 2-layer, 9-inch cake.

Best Cocoa Cake

Our best chocolate cake made with unsweetened cocoa powder—a must-try 3-layer cake.

1 cup butter or margarine
3 cups light brown sugar, lightly packed
4 eggs
2 teaspoons vanilla extract
3/4 cup unsweetened cocoa powder

3 teaspoons baking soda
1/2 teaspoon salt
3 cups sifted cake flour
1-1/3 cups dairy sour cream
1-1/3 cups boiling water

Grease and flour three 9-inch cake pans; set aside. Preheat oven to 350°F (175°C). In a large mixer bowl, cream butter or margarine until smooth. Add brown sugar and eggs. Beat with electric mixer on high speed until light and fluffy, about 5 minutes. With mixer on low speed, beat in vanilla, cocoa, baking soda and salt. Add flour alternately with sour cream, beating on low speed until smooth. Pour in boiling water; stir with spoon until blended. Pour into prepared pans. Bake 35 minutes or until done. Cool in pans 10 minutes. Turn out on wire racks. Cool completely. Frost, if desired. Makes one 3-layer, 9-inch cake.

One-Bowl Chocolate Cake

Unless you try it, you wouldn't believe a cake could be so easy and so good.

4 oz. unsweetened chocolate
2 cups sifted cake flour
2 cups sugar
1 teaspoon baking soda
1 teaspoon salt
1/2 teaspoon baking powder

3/4 cup water
3/4 cup buttermilk
1/2 cup shortening
2 eggs
1 teaspoon vanilla extract

Melt chocolate; set aside. Grease and flour two 9-inch cake pans; set aside. Preheat oven to 350°F (175°C). Combine all ingredients in a large mixer bowl. Beat with electric mixer on low speed 1/2 minute, then on high speed 3 minutes. Pour into prepared pans. Bake 30 to 35 minutes or until done. Cool in pans 5 minutes. Turn out on wire racks. Cool completely. Frost, if desired. Makes one 2-layer, 9-inch cake.

Old-Fashioned Chocolate Cake

Milk Chocolate Frosting, page 33, enhances the delicate flavor.

3/4 cup butter or margarine
1-1/2 cups sugar
3 egg yolks
1-1/2 teaspoons vanilla extract
2-1/4 cups sifted cake flour

1/2 cup unsweetened cocoa powder
3 teaspoons baking powder
1 cup cold water
3 egg whites

Grease and flour two 9-inch cake pans; set aside. Preheat oven to 350°F (175°C). In a large mixer bowl, cream butter or margarine. Gradually add sugar, creaming until light and fluffy. Add egg yolks 1 at a time, beating well after each addition. Beat in vanilla. Combine flour, cocoa and baking powder. Add to creamed mixture alternately with water, beating after each addition until smooth. In a small bowl, beat egg whites until stiff but not dry. Gently fold into batter. Pour into prepared pans. Bake about 25 minutes or until done. Cool in pans 10 minutes. Turn out on wire racks. Cool completely. Frost, if desired. Makes one 2-layer, 9-inch cake.

Marshmallow creme will spread easier if the jar is placed in a pan of hot water for a few minutes. Dipping the knife or spatula in hot water several times also makes spreading easier.

Devilish Cake

This rich, deeply colored cake is especially good with Glossy Frosting, page 32.

2 oz. unsweetened chocolate
1-3/4 cup flour
1 cup granulated sugar
1/2 cup light brown sugar, lightly packed
1-1/2 teaspoons baking soda
3/4 teaspoon salt

1-1/4 cups buttermilk
1/2 cup shortening
2 eggs
1 teaspoon vanilla extract
1/2 teaspoon red food coloring

Melt chocolate; set aside. Grease and flour two 9-inch cake pans; set aside. Preheat oven to 350°F (175°C). Combine all ingredients in a large mixer bowl. Beat with electric mixer on low speed 1/2 minute, then on high speed 3 minutes. Pour into prepared pans. Bake 30 to 35 minutes or until done. Cool in pans 10 minutes. Turn out on wire racks. Cool completely. Frost, if desired. Makes one 2-layer, 9-inch cake.

German Sweet Chocolate Cake

The authentic recipe for this famous cake—thanks to our friends at General Foods.

1 (4-oz.) pkg. Baker's German's
  Sweet Chocolate
1/2 cup boiling water
1 cup butter or margarine
2 cups sugar
4 egg yolks
1 teaspoon vanilla extract

2-1/2 cups sifted Swans Down Cake Flour
1 teaspoon baking soda
1/2 teaspoon salt
1 cup buttermilk
4 egg whites, stiffly beaten
Coconut-Pecan Frosting, see below

Coconut-Pecan Frosting:
1 cup evaporated milk
1 cup sugar
3 egg yolks, slightly beaten
1/2 cup butter or margarine

1 teaspoon vanilla extract
1-1/3 cups Baker's Angel Flake Coconut
1 cup chopped pecans

Melt chocolate in boiling water; set aside to cool. Line the bottom of three 8- or 9-inch cake pans with parchment or wax paper; set aside. Preheat oven to 350°F (175°C). Cream butter or margarine and sugar until fluffy. Add egg yolks 1 at a time, beating well after each. Blend in vanilla and chocolate-water mixture. Sift together flour, baking soda and salt. Add alternately with buttermilk to chocolate mixture, beating after each addition until smooth. Fold in beaten egg whites. Pour into prepared pans. Bake 30 to 40 minutes. Cool in pans 10 minutes. Turn out on wire racks. Cool completely. Prepare Coconut-Pecan Frosting. Frost only tops of cake layers. Makes one 3-layer 8- or 9-inch cake.

Coconut-Pecan Frosting:
Combine evaporated milk, sugar, egg yolks, butter or margarine and vanilla in a medium saucepan. Stir over medium heat until thickened, about 12 minutes. Stir in coconut and pecans. Cool, beating occasionally, until thick enough to spread.

Red Velvet Cake

An unbelievably red cake—with delicate chocolate flavor.

1/2 cup shortening

1-1/2 cups sugar

2 eggs

1 teaspoon salt

2-1/2 cups sifted cake flour

1 cup buttermilk

3 tablespoons red food coloring

2 tablespoons unsweetened cocoa powder

2 teaspoons vanilla extract

1 teaspoon baking soda

1 teaspoon vinegar

Vanilla Frosting, see below

Vanilla Frosting:

1/3 cup flour

1 cup milk

1 cup sugar

1 cup butter or margarine

1 tablespoon vanilla extract

Lightly grease and flour two 9-inch cake pans; set aside. Preheat oven to 350°F (175°C). In a large mixer bowl, cream shortening and sugar. Beat in eggs until light and fluffy. Add salt. Beat in cake flour alternately with buttermilk. Make a paste of red food coloring and cocoa. Add to batter and beat well. Mix vanilla, baking soda and vinegar in a small bowl. Sprinkle over batter and stir in. Pour into prepared pans. Bake 30 to 35 minutes or until done. Cool in pans 10 minutes. Turn out on wire racks. Cool completely. Prepare Vanilla Frosting. Frost between layers, side and top of cake. Makes one 2-layer 9-inch cake.

Vanilla Frosting:

Combine flour and milk in a small saucepan. Beat with a whisk until smooth. Stir constantly over low heat until thickened. Cool. In a medium bowl, cream sugar and butter or margarine. Add vanilla. Beat in cooled flour-milk mixture until frosting is fluffy and resembles whipped cream.

Mocha Cake

An excellent choice for your next coffee hour.

1/2 cup shortening

1 cup light brown sugar, lightly packed

3 egg yolks

1 teaspoon vanilla extract

2-1/4 cups flour

1/2 cup unsweetened cocoa powder

1-1/2 teaspoons baking soda

1/2 teaspoon salt

1-1/3 cups cold strong coffee

3 egg whites

3/4 cup granulated sugar

Grease and flour two 9-inch cake pans; set aside. Preheat oven to 350°F (175°C). In a large mixer bowl, cream shortening and brown sugar until light and fluffy. Add egg yolks 1 at a time, beating well after each addition. Stir in vanilla. Sift together flour, cocoa, baking soda and salt. Add to creamed mixture alternately with coffee, beating well after each addition. In a medium bowl, beat egg whites until soft peaks form. Gradually add granulated sugar, beating until stiff peaks form. Fold into batter. Pour into prepared pans. Bake 35 to 40 minutes or until done. Cool in pans 10 minutes. Turn out on wire racks. Cool completely. Frost. Makes one 2-layer, 9-inch cake.

How To Make
Mississippi Mud Cake

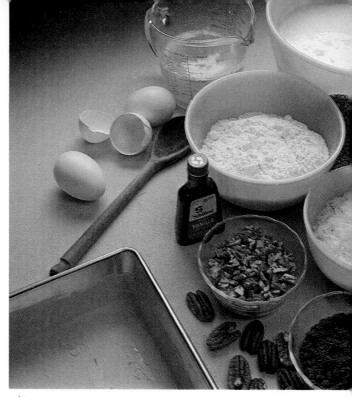

1/First, prepare the pan and measure all the ingredients.

2/As soon as you take the cake out of the oven, spread with the marshmallow creme. Heat from the freshly baked cake will soften the marshmallow.

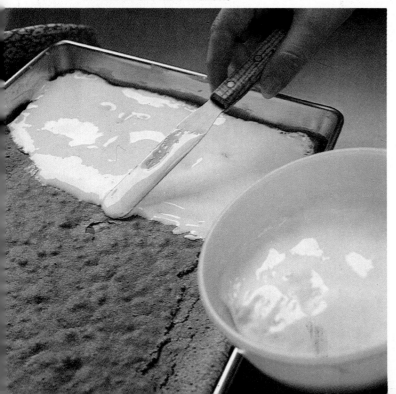

3/While marshmallow creme is still warm, gently spread frosting over the top. Then pull a spatula through both the marshmallow and frosting to make a marbled effect.

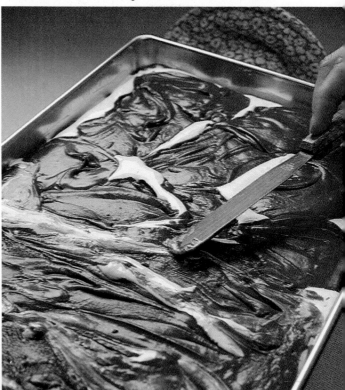

Mississippi Mud Cake

A friend of ours dislikes coconut, but that didn't stop him from downing 2 pieces of this cake!

4 eggs
2 cups sugar
1 cup butter or margarine, melted
1-1/2 cups flour
1/3 cup unsweetened cocoa powder
1 teaspoon vanilla extract

1 cup flaked coconut
1/2 cup chopped pecans
1 (7-oz.) jar marshmallow creme
Levee Frosting, see below
1 cup chopped nuts, if desired

Levee Frosting:
1/2 cup butter or margarine, melted
1/3 cup unsweetened cocoa powder
1 teaspoon vanilla extract

6 tablespoons milk
1 (1-lb.) box powdered sugar (4 cups)

Grease and flour a 13" x 9" baking pan; set aside. Preheat oven to 350°F (175°C). In a large mixer bowl, beat eggs until thick. Gradually beat in sugar. Combine melted butter or margarine with flour, cocoa, vanilla, coconut and pecans. Add to egg-sugar mixture. Stir well with a spoon. Pour into prepared pan. Bake 30 minutes or until done. Remove from oven. Immediately spread marshmallow creme gently on surface of cake. Prepare Levee Frosting. Spread frosting gently over warm marshmallow creme, swirling to give a marbled effect. Sprinkle nuts over top, if desired. Makes 1 single-layer 13" x 9" cake.

Levee Frosting:
Blend all ingredients in a medium bowl.

Banana-Nut Cake

The perfect sheet cake for a picnic.

1/3 cup butter or margarine
1-1/2 cups sugar
2 eggs
1 teaspoon vanilla extract
2 cups flour
1 teaspoon baking powder

1 teaspoon baking soda
1/2 teaspoon salt
3 tablespoons unsweetened cocoa powder
1 cup dairy sour cream
1 cup mashed ripe bananas (2 large)
1/2 cup chopped nuts

Grease a 13" x 9" baking pan; set aside. Preheat oven to 350°F (175°C). In a large mixer bowl, beat butter or margarine and sugar until light and fluffy. Beat in eggs 1 at a time. Add vanilla. Combine flour, baking powder, baking soda, salt and cocoa. Beat alternately with sour cream into creamed mixture. Stir in bananas and nuts. Pour into prepared pan. Bake 35 to 40 minutes or until done. Cool in pan. Makes 1 single-layer, 13" x 9" cake.

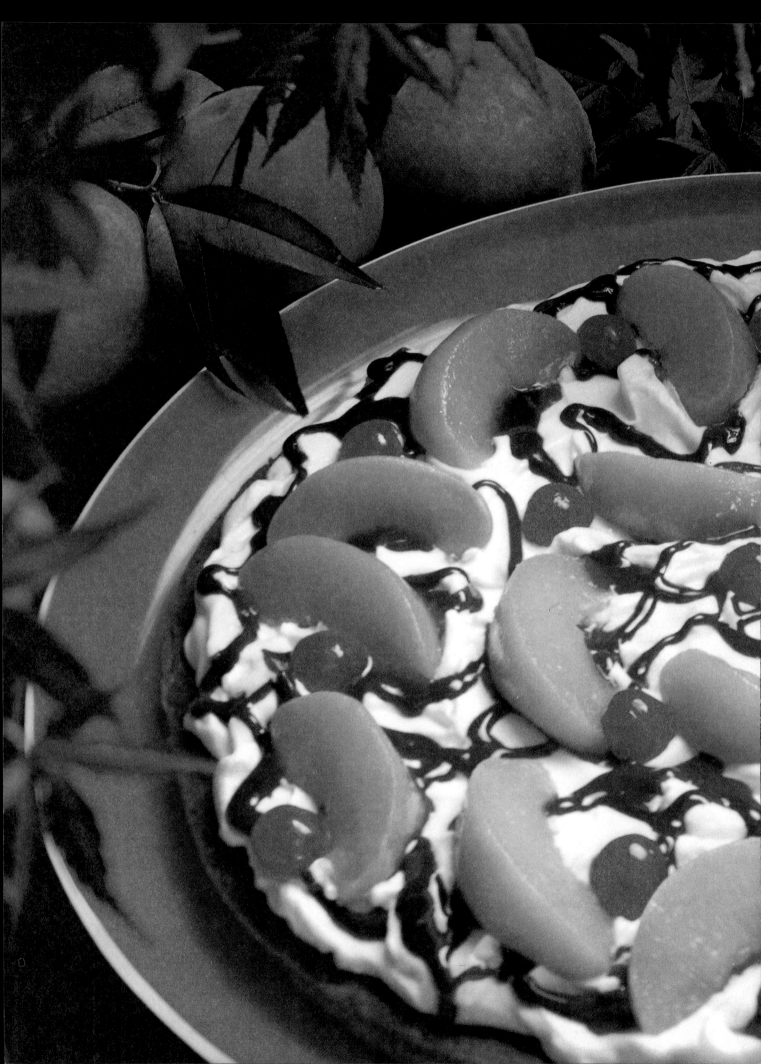

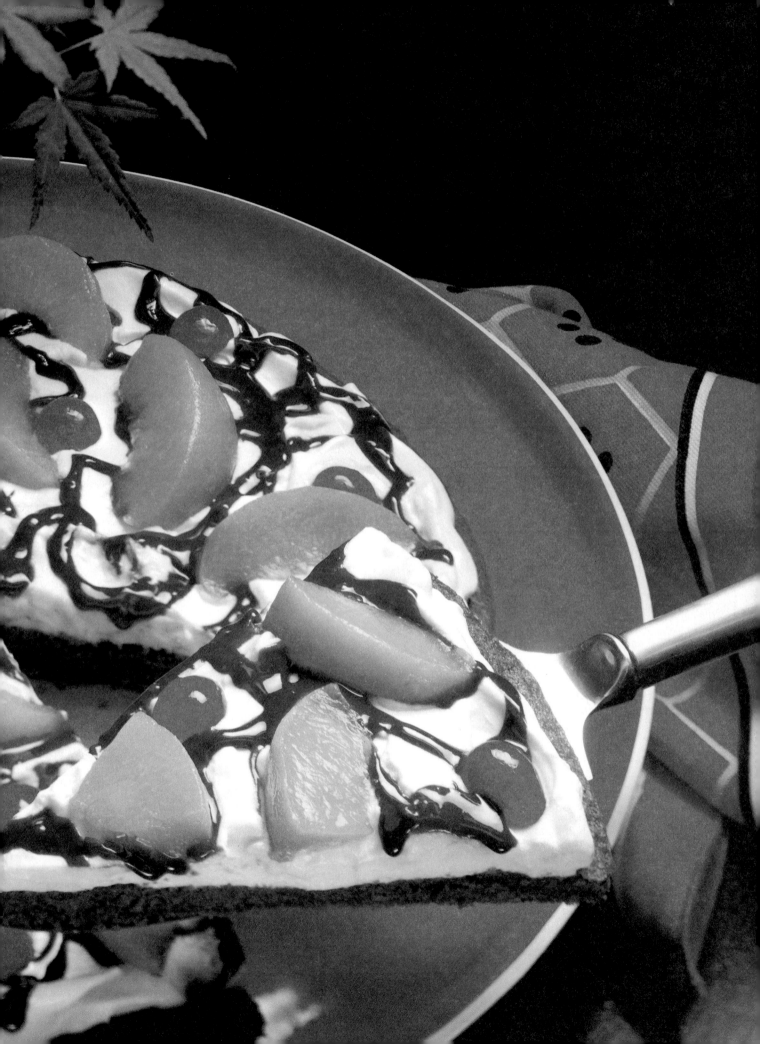

Peachy Cream Cake

A surprisingly elegant creation made in a pizza pan!

1/2 cup almond paste
3 egg yolks
1/2 cup butter or margarine
1/3 cup flour
1 teaspoon baking powder
1/2 cup chocolate syrup

3 egg whites
1 (15-oz.) can sliced peaches
1 cup whipping cream (1/2 pint)
2 tablespoons chocolate syrup
1/4 cup halved maraschino cherries

Grease and flour a 12-inch pizza pan; set aside. Preheat oven to 350°F (175°C). In a large mixer bowl, mix almond paste, egg yolks and butter or margarine. Beat until light. Mix in flour and baking powder. Add 1/2 cup chocolate syrup. In a small mixing bowl, beat egg whites until stiff. Fold into chocolate mixture. Spread batter in prepared pan. Bake 12 to 15 minutes or until done. Cool in pan. Drain peaches, reserving 1/4 cup syrup. In a small bowl, whip cream and reserved peach syrup until soft peaks form. Spread on cooled cake. Drizzle with 2 tablespoons chocolate syrup. Top with drained peaches and maraschino cherries. Cut into wedges. Makes 1 single-layer, 12-inch cake.

Peanut Butter Streusel Cake

Ideal for lunch boxes, picnics or pot lucks.

2-1/4 cups flour
2 cups light brown sugar, lightly packed
1 cup chunky peanut butter
1/2 cup butter or margarine
3 eggs
1 teaspoon baking powder

1/2 teaspoon baking soda
1 cup milk
1 teaspoon vanilla extract
1/2 cup semisweet chocolate pieces
Chocolate Glaze, see below
Chopped peanuts, if desired

Chocolate Glaze:
2 tablespoons butter or margarine
1/2 cup semisweet chocolate pieces

2 tablespoons milk
1 cup sifted powdered sugar

Grease and flour a 13" x 9" baking pan; set aside. Preheat oven to 350°F (175°C). In a large mixer bowl, combine flour and brown sugar. Mix in peanut butter and butter or margarine until mixture is crumbly. Remove 1 cup of mixture and set aside. To remaining mixture, add eggs, baking powder, baking soda, milk and vanilla. Beat with electric mixer on medium speed about 3 minutes. Spoon half of batter into prepared pan. Sprinkle with reserved cup of peanut butter mixture, then with chocolate pieces. Top with other half of cake batter. Bake 30 to 35 minutes or until done. Cool in pan. Prepare Chocolate Glaze. Spread on cooled cake. Sprinkle with peanuts, if desired. Makes 1 single-layer, 13" x 9" cake.

Chocolate Glaze:
In a small saucepan, combine butter or margarine with chocolate pieces and milk. Cook over low heat until chocolate melts. Remove from heat. Stir in powdered sugar.

Black Forest Cake

Elegant in the old world tradition.

6 eggs
1 cup sugar
1 teaspoon vanilla extract
1/2 cup flour
1/2 cup unsweetened cocoa powder
1/2 cup butter or margarine, melted

Brandied Syrup, see below
2 cups whipping cream
1/4 cup powdered sugar
1 (16-oz.) can sweet, dark pitted cherries, drained
1 oz. semisweet or milk chocolate

Brandied Syrup:
3/4 cup sugar
1 cup cold water

1/4 cup kirsch (cherry brandy) or Cointreau (orange liqueur)

Grease and flour three 8-inch cake pans; set aside. Preheat oven to 350°F (175°C). In a large mixer bowl, beat eggs until light and fluffy. Add sugar and vanilla. Beat at high speed until thick, about 5 minutes. Combine flour and cocoa in sifter. Gradually sift over egg mixture while very gently folding in. Stir in melted butter or margarine 2 tablespoons at a time until just blended. Spoon into prepared pans. Bake 15 to 20 minutes or until done. Cool in pan 5 minutes. Turn out on wire racks. Cool completely. Prepare Brandied Syrup. With a fork, prick each cake layer 12 to 14 times. Carefully spoon syrup over each layer. Whip cream until it begins to thicken. Add powdered sugar; continue beating until stiff. Place 1 cake layer on serving plate; spread with whipped cream. Top with second layer; spread with whipped cream. Place third layer on top. Arrange cherries on top layer, leaving about 1/2 inch around outer edge for whipped cream. Frost side and 1/2-inch circle on top with remaining whipped cream. Refrigerate cake. Make chocolate curls or grate chocolate with coarse side of grater. Gently press chocolate into whipped cream. Refrigerate until serving time. Makes one 3-layer, 8-inch cake.

Brandied Syrup:
In a small saucepan, bring sugar and water to a boil, stirring until sugar dissolves. Continue boiling without stirring 5 minutes. Remove from heat. Cool to lukewarm. Stir in kirsch or Cointreau.

When baking layer cakes, place pans on middle rack of oven with at least 1 inch between pans and 1 inch from sides of oven. This allows proper circulation of heat necessary for even baking.

Date Cake

A versatile dessert: serve it warm or cold, plain or with ice cream.

1 cup chopped dates
1 teaspoon grated orange peel
1 teaspoon baking soda
1-1/2 cups boiling water
3/4 cup shortening

1 cup sugar
1 egg
2 cups flour
2 teaspoons baking powder
1/2 teaspoon salt

Pecan Topping:
1/2 cup sugar
1/2 cup chopped pecans

1 (6-oz.) pkg. semisweet chocolate pieces
   (1 cup)

Grease a 13" x 9" baking pan; set aside. Preheat oven to 350°F (175°C). In a small bowl, combine dates, orange peel and baking soda. Pour boiling water over; set aside. In a large mixer bowl, cream shortening and sugar until light and fluffy. Beat in egg. Combine flour, baking powder and salt. Add alternately with date mixture to creamed mixture. Stir until blended. Pour into prepared pan. Prepare Pecan Topping. Sprinkle topping over batter in pan. Bake about 1 hour or until done.

Pecan Topping:
Mix all ingredients in a small bowl.

Spicy Fruitcake

Mellow this cake a few weeks in a brandy- or juice-soaked cloth inside a foil wrapping.

1 oz. unsweetened chocolate
1 cup currants
3 cups raisins
4 cups mixed chopped candied fruits
   and peels
1 cup pecan halves
1 cup slivered blanched almonds
2 cups flour
1 teaspoon nutmeg

1-1/2 teaspoons cinnamon
1 teaspoon ground cloves
1/2 teaspoon baking soda
1 cup shortening
1 cup light brown sugar, lightly packed
6 egg yolks
1/4 cup lemon juice
1/4 cup orange juice
6 egg whites

Melt chocolate; set aside. Grease bottom and sides of a 10-inch tube pan and line with wax paper or aluminum foil; set aside. Preheat oven to 300°F (150°C). In a large bowl, thoroughly mix currants, raisins, candied fruits and peels, nuts and 1 cup of the flour. Combine remaining flour, nutmeg, cinnamon, cloves and baking soda in a small bowl; set aside. In a large mixer bowl, cream shortening and brown sugar until light and fluffy. Add egg yolks 1 at a time, beating well after each addition. With electric mixer on low speed, blend in melted chocolate. Alternately beat in the flour-spice mixture and fruit juices, beating after each addition until just smooth. Stir into fruit-nut mixture. Beat egg whites until stiff. Fold into batter. Turn into prepared pan. Bake 2 hours and 20 minutes or until done. Cool completely in pan. Makes one 10-inch tube cake.

Chocolate Fruitcake

Chocolate fruitcake is a very special treat!

3 oz. unsweetened chocolate
1/2 cup shortening
1 cup sugar
3 eggs
2 cups flour
2 teaspoons baking powder
1 teaspoon salt

1 teaspoon cinnamon
1/3 cup milk
3 cups mixed chopped candied fruits
   and peels
1 cup raisins
1 cup chopped walnuts
1 tablespoon brandy

Grease bottom and sides of a 10-inch tube pan and line with wax paper or aluminum foil; set aside. Preheat oven to 275°F (135°C). Melt chocolate; set aside. In a large mixer bowl, cream shortening and sugar until fluffy. Add eggs 1 at a time, beating well after each addition. Stir in melted chocolate. Combine flour, baking powder, salt and cinnamon. Add to chocolate mixture alternately with milk. Stir in candied fruits and peels, raisins, walnuts and brandy. Pour into prepared pan. Bake 1 hour and 45 minutes or until done. Cool in pan 10 minutes. Turn out on wire rack. Makes one 10-inch tube cake.

Cherry-Chocolate Cake

One 9-ounce jar of maraschino cherries contains enough cherries and juice to make this.

1 oz. unsweetened chocolate
2 cups flour
1 cup sugar
1 teaspoon baking soda
1/4 teaspoon salt
1/2 cup shortening

3/4 cup milk
1/4 cup maraschino cherry juice
2 eggs
1/2 cup chopped maraschino cherries
Several drops red food coloring
Cherry-Chocolate Frosting, see below

Cherry-Chocolate Frosting:
1 oz. unsweetened chocolate
1/2 cup butter or margarine
3 cups sifted powdered sugar

1/4 cup maraschino cherry juice
1/2 cup chopped maraschino cherries

Grease and flour two 9-inch cake pans; set aside. Preheat oven to 350°F (175°C). Melt chocolate; set aside. In a large mixer bowl, combine flour, sugar, baking soda and salt. Make a well in center of flour mixture. Drop in shortening, milk, cherry juice and eggs. Blend with electric mixer on low speed, then beat on medium speed 2 minutes. Add melted chocolate, cherries and food coloring. Beat another minute. Pour into prepared pans. Bake 25 to 30 minutes or until done. Cool in pans 10 minutes. Turn out on wire racks. Cool completely. Prepare Cherry-Chocolate Frosting. Spread on cake. Makes one 2-layer, 9-inch cake.

Cherry-Chocolate Frosting:
Melt chocolate; set aside. In a small mixer bowl, cream butter or margarine. Add powdered sugar and cherry juice. Beat until smooth. Stir in melted chocolate and cherries.

Cocoa Pound Cake

Exceptionally moist and light with a mild chocolate flavor.

1 cup butter or margarine
1/2 cup shortening
3 cups sugar
5 eggs
3 cups flour

1/2 teaspoon baking powder
1/2 teaspoon salt
1/4 cup unsweetened cocoa powder
1 cup milk
1 tablespoon vanilla extract

Generously grease a 10-inch fluted tube pan; set aside. Preheat oven to 325°F (165°C). In a large mixer bowl, cream butter or margarine, shortening and sugar until light and fluffy. Add eggs 1 at a time, beating well after each addition. Combine flour, baking powder, salt and cocoa. Add alternately to creamed mixture with milk. Beat until blended. Stir in vanilla. Pour into prepared pan. Bake 1 hour and 20 minutes or until done. Cool in pan 10 minutes. Turn out on wire rack. Makes one 10-inch tube cake.

Swirled Pound Cake

You'll love the marbled effect and superb taste.

1 cup butter
2 cups sugar
6 eggs
1 cup dairy sour cream
3 teaspoons baking powder

3 cups flour
1 teaspoon vanilla extract
3 tablespoons unsweetened cocoa powder
Powdered sugar or any chocolate glaze,
   pages 30 to 40

Grease a 10-inch tube pan or a fluted tube pan; set aside. Preheat oven to 325°F (165°C). In a large mixer bowl, cream butter and sugar until light and fluffy. Add eggs 1 at a time, beating well after each addition. Mix in sour cream, baking powder, flour and vanilla. Spoon half of batter into prepared pan. Stir cocoa into remaining batter. With a large spoon, drop chocolate batter evenly on top of plain batter. Place narrow spatula down into batter and pull through both batters in a zig-zag pattern to create a marbled effect. Bake 1 hour or until done. Remove from oven. Cool in pan 10 minutes. Turn out on wire rack. When cool, sprinkle with powdered sugar or drizzle with chocolate glaze. Makes one 10-inch tube cake.

A 10-inch tube pan is what you may know as a 10-inch angel-food cake pan. A fluted tube pan is a Bundt pan, which is made in 8- or 10-inch sizes.

Cinnamon Pound Cake

Really great with ice cream!

1 cup butter	1/2 teaspoon baking soda
2 cups sugar	1/2 cup unsweetened cocoa powder
4 eggs	1 teaspoon cinnamon
2-3/4 cups flour	1 cup dairy sour cream
1/2 teaspoon baking powder	1 teaspoon vanilla extract

Grease a 10-inch tube pan; set aside. Preheat oven to 325°F (165°C). In a large mixer bowl, cream butter and sugar until smooth. Add eggs 1 at a time, beating well after each addition. Combine flour, baking powder, baking soda, cocoa and cinnamon. Add alternately to egg mixture with sour cream, beating after each addition. Stir in vanilla. Pour into prepared pan. Bake 1 hour and 15 minutes or until done. Cool in pan 10 minutes. Turn out on wire rack. Cool completely. Makes one 10-inch tube cake.

Cocoa Chiffon Cake

Just enough chocolate flavor to make it irresistible.

2 cups cake flour	7 egg yolks
1-3/4 cups sugar	3/4 cup cold water
1/3 cup unsweetened cocoa powder	1 teaspoon vanilla extract
3 teaspoons baking powder	7 egg whites
1 teaspoon salt	1/2 teaspoon cream of tartar
1/2 cup cooking oil	Creamy Glaze, see below

Creamy Glaze:

1/4 cup butter or margarine	1 teaspoon vanilla extract
2 cups sifted powdered sugar	2 tablespoons hot water

Preheat oven to 325°F (165°C). In a large mixer bowl, combine flour, sugar, cocoa, baking powder and salt. Make a well in mixture and add oil, egg yolks, water and vanilla. Beat until smooth. In another large mixer bowl, beat egg whites and cream of tartar until very stiff peaks form. Gradually pour batter over beaten whites, gently folding until just blended. Spoon into ungreased 10-inch tube pan. Bake 1 hour and 10 to 15 minutes or until done. Invert pan on wire rack. Let stand in pan upside down until completely cool. Prepare Creamy Glaze. Spoon over top of cake, letting excess drip down sides. Makes one 10-inch tube cake.

Creamy Glaze:

In a small saucepan, melt butter or margarine. Remove from heat. Stir in powdered sugar and vanilla. Add water. Mix until smooth.

Cinnamon Chiffon Cake

Delicate cinnamon and rich chocolate enhance your reputation as an accomplished cook!

2 oz. unsweetened chocolate
1 cup sugar
1-3/4 cups sifted cake flour
1/2 teaspoon salt
3/4 teaspoon baking soda
1 teaspoon cinnamon

1/3 cup cooking oil
1 cup buttermilk or sour milk
2 egg yolks
2 egg whites
1/2 cup sugar

Melt chocolate; set aside. Grease and flour two 9-inch cake pans; set aside. Preheat oven to 350°F (175°C). In a large mixer bowl, combine 1 cup sugar, flour, salt, baking soda and cinnamon. Add oil, buttermilk or sour milk and egg yolks. Beat until smooth. Stir in melted chocolate. In a small mixer bowl, beat egg whites until foamy. Gradually add 1/2 cup sugar, beating until very stiff peaks form. Gently fold beaten egg whites into chocolate mixture. Pour into prepared pans. Bake 30 to 35 minutes or until done. Cool in pans 10 minutes. Turn out on wire racks. Cool completely. Frost, if desired. Makes one 2-layer, 9-inch cake.

Chocolate Chip Chiffon Cake

Chocolate flecks lend eye appeal.

2 oz. sweet baking chocolate
2 cups flour
1-1/2 cups sugar
3 teaspoons baking powder
1/2 teaspoon salt
1/2 cup cooking oil

7 egg yolks
3/4 cup cold water
2 teaspoons vanilla extract
7 egg whites
1/2 teaspoon cream of tartar
Sweet Chocolate Glaze, see below

Sweet Chocolate Glaze:
2 oz. sweet baking chocolate
2 tablespoons butter or margarine
1 cup powdered sugar

1/2 teaspoon vanilla extract
2 tablespoons hot water

Grate chocolate; set aside. Preheat oven to 325°F (165°C). In a large mixer bowl, combine flour, sugar, baking powder and salt. Make a well in mixture and add oil, egg yolks, water and vanilla. Beat until smooth. Gently stir in grated chocolate. In another large mixer bowl, beat egg whites until foamy. Add cream of tartar; beat until very stiff peaks form. Gradually pour batter into beaten whites, folding until just blended. Pour into an ungreased, 10-inch tube pan. Bake 1 hour and 10 to 15 minutes or until done. Invert pan on cooling rack. Let stand upside down until completely cool. Prepare Sweet Chocolate Glaze. Spoon over cooled cake, letting excess drip down sides. Makes one 10-inch tube cake.

Sweet Chocolate Glaze
In a small saucepan over low heat, melt chocolate and butter or margarine. Remove from heat. Stir in powdered sugar, vanilla and hot water.

Chocolate Soufflé Roll

Peppermint-stick whipped cream wrapped in light and airy chocolate cake.

5 egg yolks
1 cup powdered sugar
1 teaspoon vanilla extract
3 tablespoons unsweetened cocoa powder
5 egg whites

1 cup whipping cream
1/3 cup finely crushed peppermint
  stick candy
Powdered sugar

Grease a 15-1/2" x 10-1/2" baking pan and line with wax paper. Grease wax paper; set aside. Preheat oven to 350°F (175°C). In a small mixer bowl, beat egg yolks until very thick and lemon-colored, 5 to 6 minutes. Gradually add powdered sugar, beating until mixture is thick again. Mix in vanilla and cocoa. In a large mixer bowl, beat egg whites until stiff but not dry. Carefully fold into egg yolk mixture. Spoon into prepared pan; spread gently and evenly. Bake 18 to 20 minutes, until done. Sprinkle a clean, dry dish towel with powdered sugar. When cake is done, remove from oven and immediately loosen sides. Invert on prepared towel. Remove wax paper. Starting with shorter edge, roll up towel and cake together. Cool rolled up cake on wire rack. When cake is cool, whip cream. Unroll cake. Remove towel. Spread cake with whipped cream. Sprinkle with crushed peppermint candy. Roll up cake like a jelly roll. Sprinkle with powdered sugar. Makes 8 servings.

Surprise Cupcakes

Use muffin pans with large cups—at least 2-1/2 inches across. Or put extra batter in lined custard cups.

1 (8-oz.) pkg. cream cheese,
  room temperature
1/3 cup sugar
1 egg
1 (6-oz.) pkg. semisweet chocolate pieces
  (1 cup)

1 (18.5-oz.) pkg. white or yellow cake mix
Liquid according to pkg. directions
Eggs according to pkg. directions

Line 24 muffin cups with fluted paper baking cups; set aside. Preheat oven to 350°F (175°C). In a medium mixing bowl, beat cream cheese with sugar and egg until smooth. Stir in chocolate pieces; set aside. Prepare cake mix according to package directions. Fill prepared muffin cups 2/3 full with cake batter. Drop a heaping teaspoon of cream cheese mixture in center of each. Cups will be almost full. Bake 15 to 20 minutes or until done. Makes 24 large cupcakes.

> *To sour milk, combine 1 tablespoon vinegar or lemon juice and enough fresh milk to make 1 cup. Let stand a few minutes before using.*

Peppermint Stick Cream Cake

An elegant dessert you can make with ease from a bakery cake.

4 oz. unsweetened chocolate	2 teaspoons vanilla extract
1 angel-food or chiffon cake	4 eggs
3/4 cup butter	1 cup whipping cream
1 cup sugar	1/4 cup crushed peppermint stick candy

Melt chocolate; set aside. Slice cake into 3 horizontal layers. In a large mixer bowl, cream butter and sugar. Beat in melted chocolate and vanilla. Add eggs 1 at a time, beating after each addition. Beat about 3 minutes or until smooth and thick. Spread chocolate mixture between cake layers and on top layer. Whip cream; fold in 2 tablespoons crushed peppermint candy. Frost sides of cake with whipped cream; sprinkle remaining candy on top. Refrigerate until serving time. Makes one 3-layer cake.

Marble Angel Cake

Delectable angel-food cake with light chocolate marbling.

6 egg yolks	1 cup sugar
12 egg whites	1 cup cake flour
1-1/2 teaspoons cream of tartar	1/4 teaspoon salt
1/2 cup sugar	2 tablespoons sweetened chocolate-flavored
1-1/2 teaspoons vanilla extract	instant cocoa mix
1/2 teaspoon almond extract	Light & Easy Glaze, see below

Light & Easy Glaze:

1 cup powdered sugar	2 tablespoons melted butter or margarine
1 tablespoon sweetened chocolate-flavored	2 tablespoons hot water
instant cocoa mix	

Preheat oven to 375°F (190°C). In a small mixer bowl, beat egg yolks with electric mixer on high speed until very thick and lemon-colored, about 5 minutes; set aside. In a large mixer bowl, beat egg whites until foamy. Add cream of tartar; beat until soft peaks form. Gradually add 1/2 cup sugar, beating until stiff peaks form. Gently fold in vanilla and almond extracts. In a medium bowl, combine 1 cup sugar, flour and salt. Sprinkle 1/4 of sugar-flour mixture over beaten egg whites; gently fold in. Repeat process until all sugar-flour mixture is folded into egg whites. Pour half the egg white mixture into another large bowl. Fold in beaten egg yolks and cocoa mix. Spoon alternate layers of white and chocolate mixtures into an ungreased 10-inch tube pan. Carefully cut through batter with a narrow spatula to create a marbled effect. Bake 40 minutes or until done. Invert on cooling rack. Let stand upside down until completely cool. Remove from pan. Prepare Light & Easy Glaze. Spoon over top of cool cake, letting excess drip down sides. Makes one 10-inch tube cake.

Light & Easy Glaze:
In a small mixer bowl, combine powdered sugar and cocoa mix. Add melted butter or margarine and hot water. Mix until smooth.

Shortcut Sicilian Cake

Start with bakery cake and finish with a superb Italian dessert.

1 (8" x 3") angel-food loaf cake
1 cup ricotta cheese
2 tablespoons sugar
1 tablespoon milk
2 tablespoons almond-flavored liqueur

1/4 cup chopped candied fruits
2 tablespoons finely chopped toasted almonds
1 oz. unsweetened chocolate, grated
Almond-Chocolate Glaze, see below

Almond-Chocolate Glaze
1/2 cup sugar
1-1/2 tablespoons cornstarch
1/2 cup water

1 oz. unsweetened chocolate, broken in chunks
1 tablespoon butter
2 teaspoons almond-flavored liqueur

Cut cake horizontally into 3 layers; set aside. In a medium mixer bowl, beat ricotta cheese, sugar, milk and liqueur until smooth. Stir in candied fruits, almonds and grated chocolate. Spread between cake layers but not on top or sides. Prepare Almond-Chocolate Glaze. Spread on top of cake, letting excess drip down sides. Refrigerate until serving time. Makes one 3-layer loaf cake.

Almond-Chocolate Glaze:
In a medium saucepan, combine sugar and cornstarch. Stir in water. Add chocolate. Stir constantly over medium heat until thickened. Remove from heat. Stir in butter and liqueur.

How To Make Marble Angel Cake

1/Create a two-toned effect by dividing beaten egg white mixture in 2 bowls. Add cocoa mix and egg yolks to one bowl. Spoon alternate layers of light and dark mixture into pan.

2/After all the mixture is in the cake pan, carefully swirl a small spatula through the batter to give a marbled effect. The top will appear slightly two-toned. When you cut the baked cake, it will have a definite marbled look.

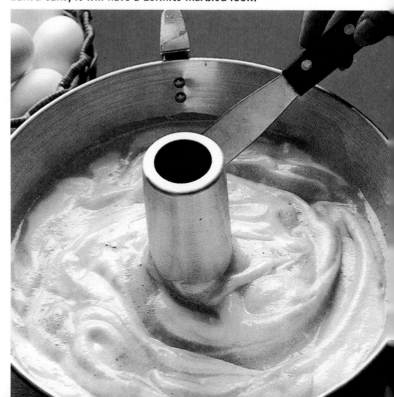

Frostings, Fillings & Sauces

As you might expect in a chocolate cookbook, most of the frostings you'll find here are made with some form of chocolate. We have included a few non-chocolate frostings just in case you like a contrast of flavors for chocolate cakes.

In a few of the cake recipes we suggested a specific frosting that we liked with that particular cake. You will find others that you might like as well or better. Next time you make a chocolate cake, look through this frosting section and match-up one that seems to go well with your cake.

Did you realize that most basic chocolate or fudge sauces can be made ahead and kept covered in the refrigerator until needed? By keeping one of these on hand, you can create an impressive dessert with ice cream or plain bakery cake at a moment's notice. For a quick hot fudge sundae, heat sauce in your microwave oven or over hot water, then spoon over ice cream and top with whipped cream and grated chocolate or chopped nuts.

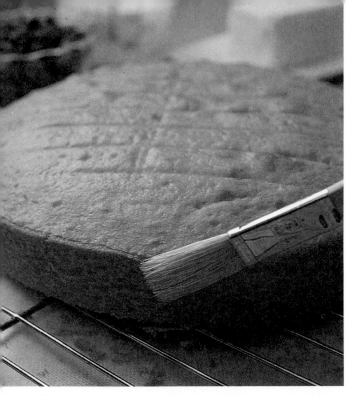

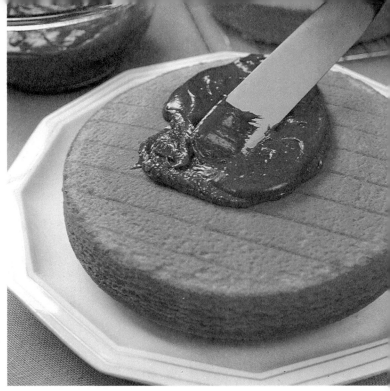

1/After layer cake is completely cooled, use your hand or a small brush to remove loose crumbs from around the sides and bottom. If these crumbs are left on the cake, they'll give the frosting a lumpy appearance.

2/Turn bottom layer of cake upside down on the plate. The flat side of the cake should be on top and the round side on the bottom. Spread frosting over this layer almost to the edge. If your recipe calls for a separate filling, spread the filling instead of the frosting between the layers.

How To Frost A Cake

3/Place second cake layer on top of frosting or filling with the bottom or flat side of this layer down and the rounded side up. This is done so the flat sides of the layers will fit together and the top will have a slight dome shape. Frost the sides of both cake layers with a thick layer of frosting. If the cake is very crumbly, first frost with a very thin layer of frosting to seal in the crumbs, then apply a thicker layer.

4/The last step is to frost the top of the cake. Spoon the remaining frosting on the top. Spread with a spatula to meet the frosting on the side. Make swirl designs or smooth the frosting with a spatula. Before the frosting sets, sprinkle with nuts, coconut or chocolate sprinkles, if desired.

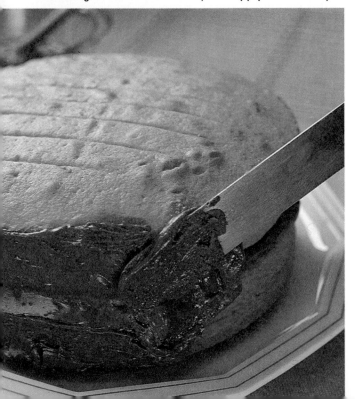

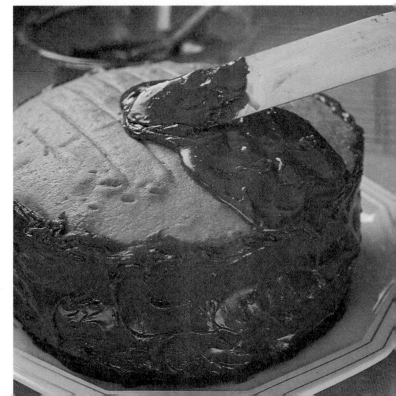

Black Beauty Frosting

Smooth, dark and creamy.

1/2 cup evaporated milk, not diluted
1/2 cup sugar
2 tablespoons butter or margarine

2 tablespoons light corn syrup
1 (6-oz.) pkg. semisweet chocolate pieces
   (1 cup)

In a medium saucepan, combine milk, sugar, butter or margarine and corn syrup. Bring to a boil, stirring constantly. Simmer 5 minutes. Remove from heat; immediately stir in chocolate pieces. Beat until smooth. Cool until spreadable. Frosts a 13" x 9" cake. Or thinly frosts the top and sides of one 2-layer, 8-inch cake.

Fudge Frosting

For a dark, rich, fudgy look.

1/4 cup butter or margarine
1 (6-oz.) pkg. semisweet chocolate pieces
   (1 cup)
1 cup granulated sugar
1/2 cup milk

1/4 teaspoon salt
2 cups powdered sugar
1 teaspoon vanilla extract
1 to 2 tablespoons milk, if needed

In a medium saucepan, combine butter or margarine with chocolate pieces, granulated sugar, milk and salt. Bring to a boil, stirring constantly. Simmer 3 minutes. Remove from heat. Stir in powdered sugar and vanilla. Beat until smooth. If frosting becomes too thick to spread, add a tablespoon or two of milk. Fills and frosts one 2-layer, 8- or 9-inch cake.

Glossy Frosting

Our favorite for Devilish Cake, page 14.

3 tablespoons shortening
3 oz. unsweetened chocolate
2 cups powdered sugar

1/4 teaspoon salt
1/3 cup milk
1 teaspoon vanilla extract

In a medium saucepan, melt shortening and chocolate over low heat. Stir in powdered sugar, salt, milk and vanilla; beat until smooth. Place saucepan in a bowl of ice water. Continue beating to spreading consistency. Fills and frosts one 2-layer, 8- or 9-inch cake.

Milk Chocolate Frosting

Cream and butter give this frosting the look and taste of milk chocolate.

1 oz. unsweetened chocolate	1 egg yolk
1/3 cup butter or margarine,	1-1/2 teaspoons vanilla extract
room temperature	2 cups sifted powdered sugar
2 cups sifted powdered sugar	About 1/4 cup light cream

Melt chocolate; set aside to cool. In a medium mixing bowl, cream butter or margarine. Gradually blend in 2 cups powdered sugar. Mix in egg yolk, melted chocolate and vanilla. Gradually beat in 2 more cups powdered sugar. Add enough cream to bring to spreading consistency. Fills and frosts one 2-layer, 8- or 9-inch cake.

Light Fudge Frosting

If you enjoy a mild and creamy fudge frosting, try this.

2 cups sugar	2 oz. unsweetened chocolate
1/4 cup light corn syrup	1/4 teaspoon salt
1/2 cup milk	1 teaspoon vanilla extract
1/2 cup shortening	

Combine all ingredients except vanilla in a medium saucepan. Stir constantly over medium heat until chocolate melts and sugar dissolves. Bring to a boil, stirring constantly. Boil rapidly, still stirring constantly, 1 minute or until mixture reaches 220°F (105°C) on a candy thermometer. Remove from heat; stir in vanilla. Place pan in a bowl of ice water to cool slightly, about 5 minutes. Beat until frosting loses its gloss and is spreadable, about 10 minutes. Fills and frosts one 2-layer 8- or 9-inch cake.

Cocoa-Butter Frosting

Quick and basic.

1/3 cup butter or margarine,	2 cups sifted powdered sugar
room temperature	1-1/2 teaspoons vanilla extract
1/3 cup unsweetened cocoa powder	3 tablespoons milk

In a medium mixing bowl, cream butter or margarine. Add cocoa, powdered sugar, vanilla and milk. Beat until frosting is smooth and spreadable. Fills and frosts one 2-layer, 8- or 9-inch cake.

Cream Cheese Frosting

Rich chocolate frosting that's ideal for a sheet cake.

2 oz. unsweetened chocolate
1 (3-oz.) pkg. cream cheese,
   room temperature

2 tablespoons milk
3-1/4 cups sifted powdered sugar
1 teaspoon vanilla extract

Melt chocolate; set aside. In a medium mixing bowl, combine cream cheese and milk. Gradually mix in powdered sugar until smooth. Add melted chocolate and vanilla. Beat until blended. Frosts 1 single-layer, 13" x 9" cake.

Sour Cream Frosting

So smooth and creamy!

1 (6-oz.) pkg. semisweet chocolate pieces
   (1 cup)
1/4 cup butter or margarine

1/2 cup dairy sour cream
1 teaspoon vanilla extract
3-1/4 cups sifted powdered sugar

In a medium saucepan, melt chocolate pieces and butter or margarine. Cool several minutes. Stir in sour cream, vanilla and powdered sugar. Beat until smooth. Fills and frosts one 2-layer, 8- or 9-inch cake.

Peanutty Frosting

Peanut butter frosting delicately flavored with chocolate and sprinkled with crunchy peanuts.

2 oz. semisweet chocolate
2 tablespoons butter or margarine,
   room temperature
2 tablespoons peanut butter

1 teaspoon vanilla extract
3 cups powdered sugar
5 tablespoons milk
Chopped peanuts

Melt chocolate; set aside. In a medium bowl, cream butter or margarine and peanut butter. Stir in melted chocolate and vanilla. Add powdered sugar alternately with milk, beating until creamy and smooth. Sprinkle top of frosted cake with chopped peanuts. Fills and frosts one 2-layer, 8- or 9-inch cake.

Mint Frosting

Easy-to-make fluffy mint frosting is a natural for chocolate cakes.

2 egg whites
1/4 cup sugar
1/8 teaspoon salt

3/4 cup light corn syrup
1/4 teaspoon peppermint extract
Several drops red food coloring

In a small mixer bowl, beat egg whites until foamy. Gradually add sugar and salt; beat until stiff peaks form. In a small saucepan, heat corn syrup to boiling. Slowly pour hot corn syrup over beaten egg whites, beating constantly. Add peppermint extract and food coloring. Continue beating until thick enough to spread. Fills and frosts one 2-layer, 8- or 9-inch cake.

Mocha Frosting

A popular blend of cocoa and coffee.

1/4 cup butter or margarine,
   room temperature
2-1/2 cups sifted powdered sugar

2 tablespoons unsweetened cocoa powder
1 teaspoon vanilla extract
2 tablespoons hot strong coffee

In a medium mixing bowl, cream butter or margarine. Add powdered sugar gradually, beating constantly. Mix in cocoa, vanilla and coffee. Beat until smooth. Fills and frosts one 2-layer, 8- or 9-inch cake.

Marshmallow Frosting

This deluxe frosting is worth the extra beating.

2 egg whites
1-1/2 cups sugar
1/4 teaspoon cream of tartar

1 tablespoon light corn syrup
1/3 cup water
1-1/2 cups miniature marshmallows

In top of a double boiler, combine egg whites, sugar, cream of tartar, corn syrup and water. Beat with electric mixer on low speed for 1 minute. Place over boiling water. Beat on high speed until stiff peaks form or about 7 minutes. Remove from heat. Add marshmallows. Continue beating until frosting will spread easily. Fills and frosts one 3-layer, 8- or 9-inch cake.

Rich Vanilla Frosting

Melt-in-your-mouth vanilla frosting with chocolate cake is a terrific flavor contrast.

1-1/2 cups milk
1/2 cup flour
1-1/2 cups butter or margarine,
   room temperature

1-1/2 cups sugar
1 tablespoon vanilla extract

In a small saucepan, combine milk and flour. Beat with a wire whisk or rotary beater until smooth. Cook over low heat until thick; cool. In a medium mixing bowl, cream butter or margarine and sugar until light and fluffy. Beating with electric mixer on high speed, gradually add milk-flour mixture. Beat until smooth. Stir in vanilla. Fills and frosts one 3-layer, 8- or 9-inch cake.

Vanilla Butter Frosting

Basic creamy vanilla frosting emphasizes your favorite chocolate cake.

1/2 cup butter or margarine,
   room temperature
1 (1-lb.) box powdered sugar (4 cups)

2 teaspoons vanilla extract
3 tablespoons milk
1 to 2 tablespoons milk, if needed

Blend butter or margarine and powdered sugar in a medium mixing bowl. Stir in vanilla and milk. Beat until smooth, thick and creamy. If necessary, add 1 to 2 teaspoons milk to make frosting spreadable. Frosts one 2-layer, 8- or 9-inch cake.

Royal Chocolate Sauce

The king of chocolate sauces!

1/2 cup light corn syrup
1 cup sugar
1 cup water
3 oz. unsweetened chocolate,
   broken in chunks

1 teaspoon vanilla extract
1/2 cup evaporated milk, not diluted

In a small saucepan, combine corn syrup, sugar and water. Cook over medium-low heat to 236°F (113°C) on a candy thermometer or to soft-ball stage. Remove from heat. Stir in chocolate until melted. Add vanilla. Gradually add evaporated milk, stirring constantly until blended. Cool. Serve over ice cream or cake. Makes 1-2/3 cups sauce.

Hot Fudge Sauce

Don't eat it all at once! Store extra in the refrigerator for tomorrow.

1 (13-oz.) can evaporated milk, not diluted
2 cups sugar
4 oz. unsweetened chocolate

1/4 cup butter or margarine
1 teaspoon vanilla extract
1/2 teaspoon salt

Bring milk and sugar to a rolling boil over medium-low heat, stirring constantly. Boil and stir 1 minute longer. Add chocolate; stir until melted. Beat over heat until smooth. If sauce has a curdled appearance, beat vigorously with a wire whisk or rotary beater until creamy smooth. Remove from heat. Blend in butter or margarine, vanilla and salt. Cool to lukewarm. Serve over ice cream. Makes 3 cups sauce.

Chocolate Chip Sauce

Quick as a wink to make!

1 (6-oz.) pkg. semisweet chocolate pieces
　(1 cup)
1/2 cup light corn syrup

1/4 cup milk
1 tablespoon butter or margarine
1/4 teaspoon vanilla extract

In a small saucepan, combine all ingredients. Stir constantly over low heat until blended and smooth. Cool. Serve over ice cream or cake. Makes 1-1/4 cups sauce.

Fudge Sauce

Be sure you're melting the chocolate over very low heat.

2 oz. unsweetened chocolate
1 tablespoon butter or margarine
1/3 cup boiling water

1 cup sugar
2 tablespoons light corn syrup
1 teaspoon vanilla extract

In a small saucepan, over very low heat, melt chocolate with butter or margarine, stirring constantly. Add boiling water, sugar and corn syrup, stirring until sugar dissolves. Increase heat to medium-low. Simmer 4 minutes without stirring. Stir in vanilla. Cool to lukewarm. Serve over ice cream or cake. Makes 1-1/8 cups sauce.

Mallow-Mint Sauce

Airy chocolate sauce with a light mint flavor.

4 oz. sweet cooking chocolate,
   broken in chunks
2/3 cup evaporated milk, not diluted

8 large marshmallows
10 buttermints, crushed (1/4 cup)

In a small saucepan, combine chocolate, milk and marshmallows. Stir over very low heat until chocolate melts. Remove from heat. Mix in crushed mints. Serve warm or cold. Makes 1-1/2 cups sauce.

Fudgy Mint Sauce

Serve ice cream or cake with a cordial touch.

1/2 cup sugar
1/2 cup water
2 tablespoons light corn syrup
2 tablespoons butter or margarine

1 (6-oz.) pkg. semisweet chocolate pieces
   (1 cup)
2 tablespoons crème de menthe

In a small saucepan, combine sugar, water, corn syrup and butter or margarine. Bring to a boil over moderate heat, stirring constantly. Simmer 3 minutes. Remove from heat. Immediately add chocolate pieces. Beat with a wire whisk or rotary beater. Stir in crème de menthe. Serve warm or cool, over ice cream or cake. Makes about 1-1/2 cups sauce.

Mocha Sauce

Just right for pouring over desserts.

1/4 cup unsweetened cocoa powder
1/2 cup strong coffee

1/2 cup honey
1/4 cup whipping cream

In a small saucepan, combine cocoa, coffee, honey and cream. Stir constantly over low heat until slightly thickened and smooth. Cool. Serve over ice cream, angel-food cake or cream puffs. Makes 1 cup sauce.

Cream Filling

Creamy texture, mild chocolate flavor and light chocolate color.

1/2 cup sugar
1/4 cup flour
1 cup milk
1 egg, slightly beaten

1 oz. pre-melted unsweetened
   baking chocolate
1 teaspoon vanilla extract

In a small saucepan, combine sugar and flour. Stir in milk. Stir constantly over low heat until smooth and thickened. Remove from heat. Stir a small amount of hot mixture into egg. Add egg mixture to remaining hot mixture in saucepan. Mix in chocolate. Stir constantly over very low heat 1 minute longer. Remove from heat. Stir in vanilla. Cover and chill. Use as filling for layer cake or jelly roll. Makes about 1-1/2 cups filling.

Grasshopper Filling

This easy filling will impress your most discriminating guests.

1/4 cup crème de menthe
1 (7 oz.) jar marshmallow creme

1/2 pint whipping cream (1 cup)
Several drops green food coloring

In a medium bowl, stir crème de menthe into marshmallow creme. Whip cream in a small bowl, Fold whipped cream and food coloring into marshmallow mixture. Use as a filling for chocolate cups, jelly roll, chocolate cakes or baked meringues. Makes 3-1/2 cups filling.

Fluffy Filling

Perfect for layer cakes, cream puffs or éclairs.

1 (6-oz.) pkg. semisweet chocolate pieces
   (1 cup)
1/2 cup butter or margarine,
   room temperature

2/3 cup powdered sugar
2 egg yolks
1 teaspoon vanilla extract
2 egg whites

Melt chocolate pieces; set aside. In a medium bowl, cream butter or margarine and powdered sugar until light and fluffy. Add egg yolks 1 at a time, beating after each addition. Gradually beat in melted chocolate and vanilla. In a small bowl, beat egg whites until stiff but not dry. Fold into chocolate mixture. Use as filling for cakes, cream puffs or éclairs. Makes about 2 cups filling.

Almond Glaze

After you've glazed a favorite cake, sprinkle the top with chopped toasted almonds.

1 cup sugar
3 tablespoons cornstarch
1 cup water

2 oz. unsweetened chocolate, broken in chunks
3 tablespoons butter or margarine
1 tablespoon almond-flavored liqueur

In a medium saucepan, combine sugar and cornstarch. Stir in water. Add chocolate. Stir constantly over medium heat until thickened. Remove from heat; stir in butter or margarine and liqueur. Makes glaze for top of one 2-layer, 8- or 9-inch cake or torte.

Hurry-Up Glaze

You don't have to wait for the chocolate to melt—you buy it that way!

1 oz. pre-melted unsweetened
  baking chocolate
1 cup sifted powdered sugar

1/4 cup melted butter or margarine
2 tablespoons boiling water

In a small bowl, combine chocolate and powdered sugar. Mix in melted butter or margarine and boiling water. Stir until smooth. Makes glaze for top of one 8- or 9-inch cake or torte.

How To Glaze A Cake

1/Place cooled cake upside down on cake plate. Use your hand or small brush to remove loose crumbs from side and top. Spoon glaze over top of cake. Spread glaze evenly with back of spoon or with a small spatula.

2/Spread a small amount of glaze over edges of cake. A very thin glaze will drip over the side and down to the plate. A thicker glaze may be spread over top and sides with a spatula. Many glazes set up fast, so work quickly. If glaze becomes too thick, stir in a few drops of milk or water.

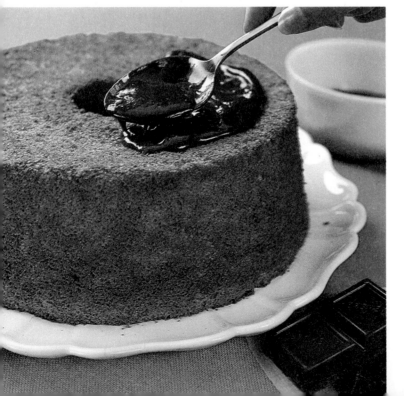

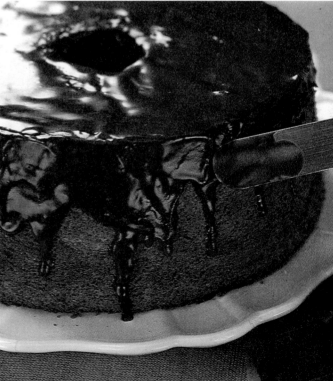

Bars & Cookies

Our cookie section is loaded with all kinds of goodies just brimming with chocolate! Especially irresistible is our collection of brownies and other bar-type cookies. If you like to make drop cookies, you'll find such favorites as Crinkles and Sour Cream Cookies. Cookie-makers who like the challenge of specially shaped treats will be tempted by Acorn Cookies and Pretzel Cookies.

You'll notice that chocolate appears in many forms in these cookies. Be sure to use the kind of chocolate indicated in the recipe. If a recipe calls for either semisweet or milk chocolate pieces, with no mention of melting the chocolate, you will be stirring the little teardrop-shaped pieces into the cookie batter. They soften in the baking process but do not melt. The tiny pieces of chocolate retain their original size and shape. On the other hand, if the recipe calls for melted chocolate, you can follow directions for melting chocolate on pages 4 and 5, then stir the melted chocolate into the batter. When baked, the whole cookie will be a chocolate color.

Although you can re-use the same cookie sheet for baking the drop-type and shaped cookies, you can hurry the baking process by using two or more cookie sheets. While one sheet of cookies is baking, you can be getting another ready for the oven. Be sure to let the pans cool before placing the uncooked dough on them. Also, cookie dough spreads when baked, so don't place the cookies too close together on the cookie sheet.

Chopped pecans and walnuts are interchangeable in most cookie doughs. Use your favorite or whichever is the most economical at the time.

Fudge Brownies

Our favorite brownie!

1/4 cup butter or margarine

2 oz. unsweetened chocolate

2 eggs

1 cup sugar

1/4 teaspoon salt

1/2 teaspoon vanilla extract

1/2 cup flour

1/2 cup chopped nuts

In a small saucepan, melt butter or margarine and chocolate over low heat; set aside to cool. Preheat oven to 350°F (175°C). In a medium mixing bowl, beat eggs until light and foamy. Beat in sugar. Add salt and vanilla. Stir in cooled chocolate mixture, then stir in flour. Fold in nuts. Bake in an ungreased 8-inch square pan about 20 minutes or until edges begin to leave side of pan. Cool in pan before cutting. Makes 16 brownies.

Hazel's Brownies

Great for picnics or lunchboxes.

3/4 cup butter or margarine, melted

1-1/2 cups sugar

1 teaspoon vanilla extract

1/4 teaspoon salt

3 eggs

1/2 cup unsweetened cocoa powder

3/4 teaspoon baking powder

1 cup flour

1/2 cup chopped nuts

Butter a 9-inch square baking pan; set aside. Preheat oven to 350°F (175°C). In a large mixer bowl, combine melted butter or margarine and sugar. Beat until blended. Add vanilla, salt and eggs. Beat well. Add cocoa, baking powder and flour, mixing until smooth. Stir in nuts. Pour into prepared pan. Bake 25 to 30 minutes. Cool in pan before cutting. Makes 16 to 20 brownies.

Peanut Butter Brownies

Easy peanutty squares with strong chocolate flavor.

2 oz. unsweetened chocolate

1/4 cup butter or margarine

1/4 cup peanut butter

1 cup light brown sugar, lightly packed

2 eggs

1 teaspoon vanilla extract

1/2 cup flour

1/2 cup chopped peanuts

Melt chocolate; set aside to cool. Grease an 8-inch square pan; set aside. Preheat oven to 325°F (165°C). In a medium mixing bowl, cream butter or margarine, peanut butter and brown sugar. Beat in eggs and vanilla. Mix in melted chocolate, then flour. Stir in peanuts. Pour into prepared pan. Bake 30 to 35 minutes or until edges begin to leave sides of pan. Cool in pan before cutting. Makes 16 brownies.

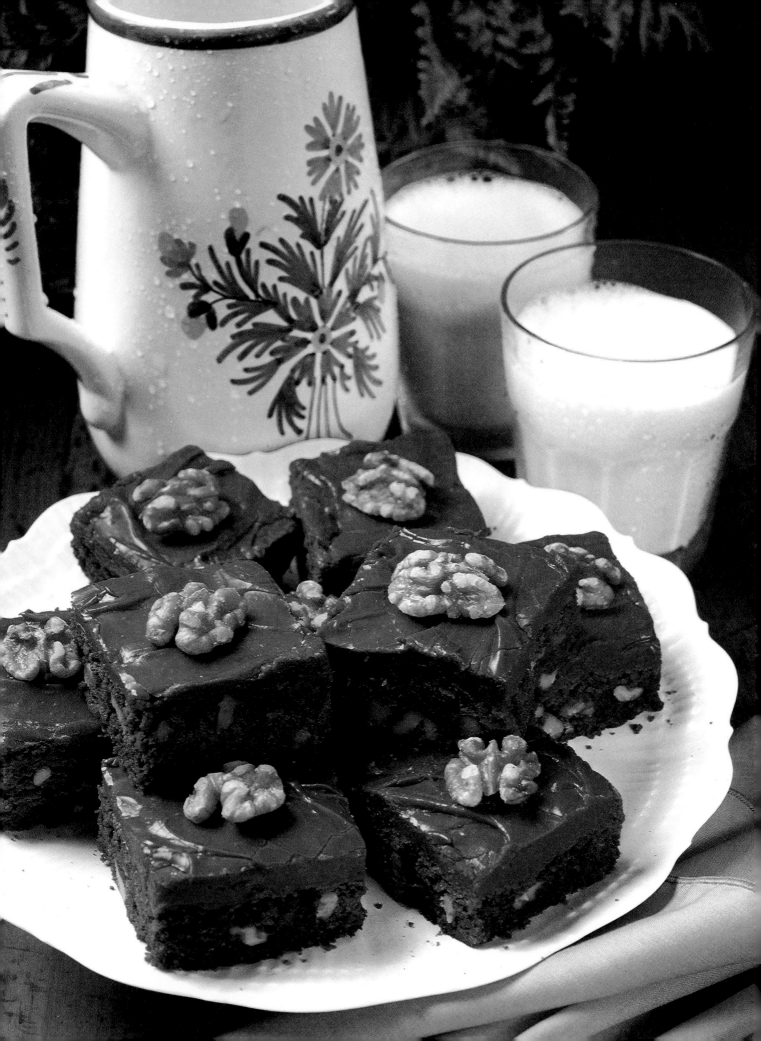

Cream Cheese Brownies

The little extra preparation time is worth this fantastic treat!

3 tablespoons butter or margarine
4 oz. sweet cooking chocolate
2 tablespoons butter or margarine,
   room temperature
1 (3-oz.) pkg. cream cheese,
   room temperature
1/4 cup sugar
1 egg
1 tablespoon flour

1 teaspoon vanilla extract
2 eggs
3/4 cup sugar
1/2 cup flour
1/2 teaspoon baking powder
1/2 teaspoon salt
1/2 cup chopped walnuts
1 teaspoon vanilla extract
1/4 teaspoon almond extract

In top of a double boiler over hot water, melt 3 tablespoons butter or margarine and chocolate. Remove from hot water; set aside to cool. Grease a 9-inch square baking pan; set aside. Preheat oven to 350°F (175°C). In a medium mixing bowl, cream 2 tablespoons butter or margarine with cream cheese until fluffy. Beat in 1/4 cup sugar, 1 egg, 1 tablespoon flour and 1 teaspoon vanilla; set aside. In a large mixer bowl, beat 2 eggs until foamy. Add 3/4 cup sugar; continue beating until blended. Stir in 1/2 cup flour, baking powder and salt. Stir in melted chocolate mixture, walnuts, 1 teaspoon vanilla and almond extract. Spread half of chocolate batter evenly in prepared pan. Spread cream cheese mixture on top. Drop spoonfuls of remaining chocolate mixture on top of cream cheese mixture. Swirl top of batter slightly with a fork. Bake 40 to 50 minutes or until edges begin to leave sides of pan. Cool in pan before cutting. Makes 16 brownies.

Swirled Mint Brownies

A double taste-treat for a new brownie experience.

3/4 cup shortening
1 cup sugar
3 eggs
1 cup flour
3/4 teaspoon baking powder

1/4 teaspoon salt
1/4 cup chocolate syrup
1/2 teaspoon peppermint extract
Several drops red food coloring

Preheat oven to 350°F (175°C). Grease a 13" x 9" baking pan. In a medium mixer bowl, cream shortening and sugar until fluffy. Beat in eggs. Combine flour, baking powder and salt. Stir into creamed mixture. Spoon half the batter into another bowl. Stir chocolate syrup into remaining batter. To the other half of batter, add peppermint extract and enough food coloring to make a medium pink mixture. Drop each mixture by rounded tablespoonfuls into prepared pan, alternating the chocolate and mint batters in a checkerboard pattern. Gently swirl spatula through checkerboard in a ziz-zag pattern to create a marbled effect. Bake 22 to 25 minutes. Cool in pan before cutting. Serve plain or frosted. Makes about 32 brownies.

Peanut Butter Dreams

An exquisite blend of chocolate and coconut over a peanut butter crust.

1/2 cup peanut butter
1/4 cup butter or margarine,
    room temperature

1/2 cup light brown sugar, lightly packed
1 cup flour
Coconut-Chocolate Topping, see below

Coconut-Chocolate Topping:
2 eggs
1 cup light brown sugar, lightly packed
1 teaspoon vanilla extract
2 tablespoons flour
1 teaspoon baking powder

1/2 teaspoon salt
3/4 cup flaked or shredded coconut
1 (6-oz.) pkg. semisweet chocolate pieces
    (1 cup)

Preheat oven to 350°F (175°C). In a medium mixing bowl, blend peanut butter, butter or margarine and brown sugar. Stir in flour. Turn out into an ungreased 13" x 9" baking pan. Flatten dough with hand to cover bottom of pan. Bake 10 minutes. While baking, prepare Coconut-Chocolate Topping. Spread topping on baked crust. Return to oven; bake 25 minutes or until golden brown. Cool slightly in pan before cutting into 1" x 3" bars. Makes about 39 bars.

Coconut-Chocolate Topping:

In a medium mixing bowl, beat eggs well. Add brown sugar and vanilla. Beat until blended. Mix in flour, baking powder and salt. Stir in coconut and chocolate pieces.

Oven S'Mores

Candy bar pieces and marshmallow creme sandwiched between crisp golden brown layers.

1/2 cup butter or margarine,
    room temperature
3/4 cup sugar
1 egg
1 teaspoon vanilla extract

1-1/2 cups flour
1/4 teaspoon salt
1 teaspoon baking powder
3 (1.05-oz.) milk chocolate candy bars
1 (7-oz.) jar marshmallow creme

Grease an 8-inch square baking pan. Preheat oven to 350°F (175°C). In a large mixer bowl, cream butter or margarine and sugar until light and fluffy. Beat in egg and vanilla. Add flour, salt and baking powder. Beat until well-mixed. Pat half of dough in bottom of prepared pan. Break candy bars into squares. Arrange squares over dough. Spread with marshmallow creme. Drop remaining dough over filling in small patches. If possible, gently spread over marshmallow. Bake 25 to 30 minutes or until golden brown. Cool in pan before cutting. Makes 16 squares.

Cherry-Chocolate Bars

A no-fuss quickie for the holidays.

2 cups finely crushed graham cracker crumbs
   (about 20 crackers)
1 (6-oz.) pkg. semisweet chocolate pieces
   (1 cup)

1 (14-oz.) can sweetened condensed milk
1/2 cup flaked coconut
1/2 cup chopped nuts
1/2 cup chopped candied cherries

Grease an 8-inch square baking pan; set aside. Preheat oven to 350°F (175°C). In a medium bowl, combine graham cracker crumbs, chocolate pieces, milk, coconut, nuts and cherries. Spoon into prepared pan. Bake 25 to 30 minutes. Cool in pan before cutting. Makes 16 squares.

Butterscotch Bars

Cornflakes add a crunchy surprise to these satisfying bars.

1-1/3 cups flour
1/2 cup light brown sugar, lightly packed
2/3 cup butter or margarine
1 cup granulated sugar
1 cup light corn syrup

1 (6-oz.) pkg. butterscotch pieces (1 cup)
1 (12-oz.) jar peanut butter (about 1-1/2 cups)
3 cups cornflakes
Creamy Chocolate Frosting, see below

Creamy Chocolate Frosting:
1/2 cup semisweet chocolate pieces
2 tablespoons butter or margarine
1 tablespoon milk

1/4 cup powdered sugar
1/2 teaspoon vanilla extract

Preheat oven to 350°F (175°C). In a small mixer bowl, blend flour, brown sugar and butter or margarine with electric mixer on low speed. Mixture will be crumbly. Pat in bottom of an ungreased 13" x 9" baking pan. Bake 15 to 20 minutes. While baking, bring granulated sugar and corn syrup to a boil in a large saucepan over medium heat, stirring occasionally. Remove from heat. Add butterscotch pieces and peanut butter. Stir until melted. Stir in cornflakes. Spread over baked crust. Cool. Prepare Creamy Chocolate Frosting. Frost cooled cake before cutting into 1" x 3" bars. Makes 39 bars.

Creamy Chocolate Frosting:
Combine chocolate pieces, butter or margarine and milk in a small saucepan. Place over low heat until chocolate and butter or margarine are melted. Remove from heat. Add powdered sugar and vanilla. Mix well.

From top to bottom: Pecan Rounds, page 54, Cherry-Chocolate Bars, page 46, Acorn Cookies, page 58, and Spritz Cookies, page 56

46

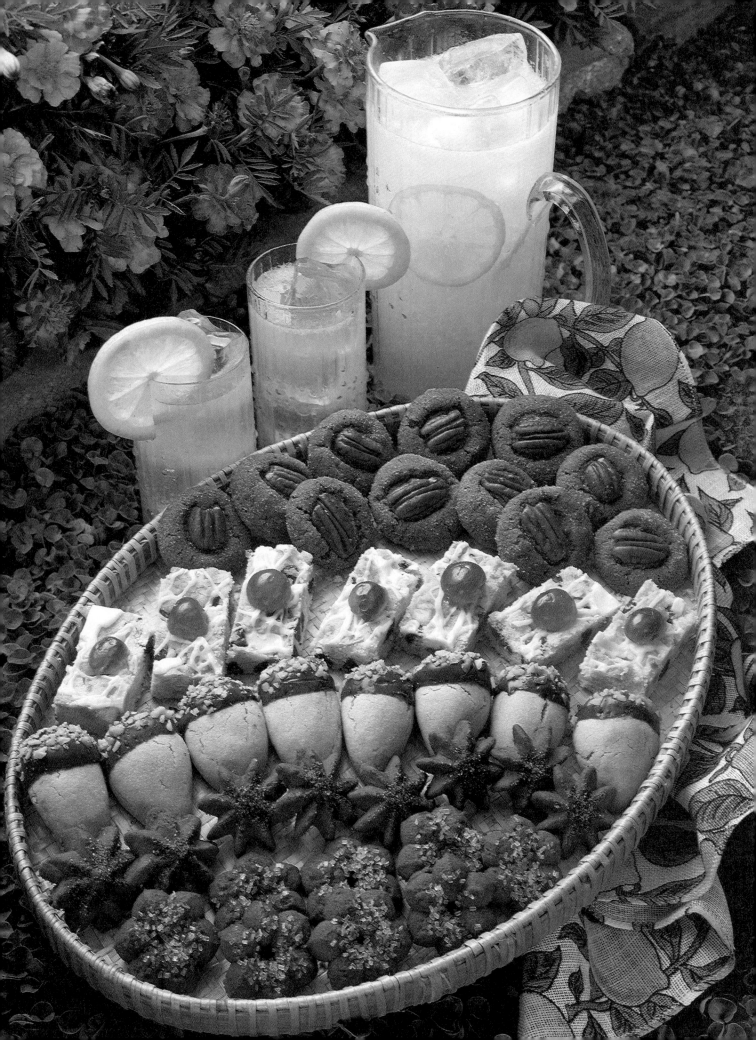

Granola Bars

Make your own and keep them on hand for a quick breakfast or snack.

1/4 cup butter or margarine
1/4 cup shortening
1 cup light brown sugar, lightly packed
1 egg
1 teaspoon vanilla extract
1-1/3 cups flour
1/2 teaspoon baking soda
1/2 teaspoon salt

1/2 teaspoon cinnamon
1/4 cup milk
1-2/3 cups granola cereal
1 cup raisins
1 cup flaked coconut
1 (6-oz.) pkg. semisweet chocolate pieces
   (1cup)

Line a 15-1/2" x 10-1/2" x 1" jelly roll pan with aluminum foil; set aside. Preheat oven to 350°F (175°C). In a large mixer bowl, cream butter or margarine, shortening, brown sugar, egg and vanilla. Combine flour, baking soda, salt and cinnamon. Add alternately with milk to creamed mixture. Stir in cereal, raisins, coconut and chocolate pieces. Spread batter evenly in prepared pan. Bake 20 to 25 minutes or until done. Cool in pan completely. Invert pan and remove. Peel off foil. Cut into bars. Makes 70 bars.

Spicy Apple-Peanut Bars

Deliciously compatible flavors!

1/3 cup shortening, room temperature
3/4 cup sugar
2 eggs
3/4 cup flour
3/4 teaspoon baking powder
1/2 teaspoon baking soda
1/2 teaspoon salt
1 tablespoon unsweetened cocoa powder

1 teaspoon cinnamon
1/2 teaspoon nutmeg
1/4 teaspoon ground cloves
1 cup uncooked rolled oats
1-1/2 cups diced peeled apple
1/2 cup chopped peanuts
Powdered sugar

Lightly grease a 9-inch square baking pan; set aside. Preheat oven to 375°F (190°C). In a large mixer bowl, cream shortening and sugar until light and fluffy. Add eggs 1 at a time, beating until very light and fluffy. Combine flour, baking powder, baking soda, salt, cocoa, cinnamon, nutmeg and cloves. With electric mixer on low speed, beat flour mixture into egg mixture until just combined. Stir in oats, apple and peanuts. Turn mixture into prepared pan. Bake 25 minutes or until edges begin to leave sides of pan. Cool completely before cutting. Sprinkle with powdered sugar. Makes 18 bars.

Butter Pecan Turtles

Tastes like those delicious turtle candies.

1-1/2 cups flour
3/4 cup light brown sugar, lightly packed
1/3 cup butter or margarine,
   room temperature

1/2 cup chopped pecans
1/2 cup butter or margarine
1/3 cup light brown sugar, lightly packed
1 cup milk chocolate pieces

Preheat oven to 350°F (175°). Place flour and 3/4 cup brown sugar in a medium mixing bowl. With pastry blender or fork, cut in 1/3 cup butter or margarine until crumbly and well-mixed. Pat firmly on bottom of an ungreased 9-inch square baking pan. Sprinkle pecans over top. In a small saucepan, bring 1/2 cup butter or margarine and 1/3 cup brown sugar to a boil. Simmer 1 minute, stirring constantly. Remove from heat. Gently pour over pecans, covering all crust if possible. Bake 15 to 20 minutes or until caramel is bubbly over entire top. Remove from oven. Immediately sprinkle with chocolate pieces. Let stand to slightly melt chocolate. Gently swirl spatula through caramel and chocolate to create a marbled effect. Cool in pan before cutting. Makes 24 to 27 bars.

Rocky Road Bars

Scrumptious melted marshmallows and chocolate topping over nutty chocolate bars.

1/3 cup butter or margarine
1 oz. unsweetened chocolate
1 cup sugar
2 eggs, beaten
3/4 cup flour
1/2 teaspoon salt

1/2 teaspoon baking powder
1 teaspoon vanilla extract
1/2 cup chopped pecans
16 large marshmallows, halved
Chocolate Topping, see below

Chocolate Topping:
2 oz. unsweetened chocolate
1/4 cup butter or margarine
2 cups powdered sugar

1/4 cup milk
1 teaspoon vanilla extract

Grease an 11" x 7" baking pan; set aside. Preheat oven to 350°F (175°C). Melt butter or margarine and chocolate over low heat. Remove from heat. Beat in sugar, then eggs. Combine flour, salt and baking powder. Stir into chocolate mixture. Add vanilla and pecans. Pour into prepared pan. Bake 35 minutes. Remove from oven. Immediately top with marshmallows. Return to oven for 3 minutes or until marshmallows are soft. Set aside while preparing Chocolate Topping. Pour topping over warm marshmallows. Cool in pan before cutting. Makes 33 bars.

Chocolate Topping:
Combine chocolate and butter or margarine in a small saucepan. Place over low heat until just melted. Combine powdered sugar, milk and vanilla in a small mixer bowl. Add chocolate mixture. Beat until smooth.

Crunchy Almond Bars

Lots of crunch appeal—and pretty, too.

1 cup shortening
1-1/4 cups sugar
1 egg
1/4 teaspoon almond extract
2-1/4 cups flour
1/2 teaspoon baking powder
1-1/2 teaspons salt

1/2 cup toasted slivered almonds
1/2 cup candied cherries, halved
1/2 cup flaked coconut
1 (6-oz.) pkg. semisweet chocolate pieces
   (1 cup)
Simply Sweet Glaze, see below
Sliced candied cherries for garnish

Simply Sweet Glaze:
1 tablespoon butter or margarine
1 tablespoon milk

1 cup sifted powdered sugar

Grease a 16" x 11" baking pan. Set aside. Preheat oven to 375°F (190°C). In a large mixer bowl, cream shortening and sugar until light and creamy. Beat in egg and almond extract. Add flour, baking powder and salt. Mix well. Stir in almonds, candied cherries, coconut and chocolate pieces. Spread in prepared pan. Bake 20 minutes. Cool slightly. While baking, prepare Simply Sweet Glaze. Drizzle glaze over warm cake. Cut into 1" x 2" bars. Garnish each bar with a cherry slice. Makes about 70 bars.

Simply Sweet Glaze:
In a small saucepan, melt butter or margarine with milk over low heat. Remove from heat. Stir in powdered sugar until creamy.

Original Toll House® Cookies

Cookies made with this traditional recipe disappear on the way to the cookie jar!

2-1/4 cups flour
1 teaspoon baking soda
1 teaspoon salt
1 cup butter or margarine,
   room temperature
3/4 cup granulated sugar

3/4 cup brown sugar, firmly packed
1 teaspoon vanilla extract
2 eggs
1 (12-oz.) pkg. Nestlé Semi-Sweet
   Real Chocolate Morsels (2 cups)
1 cup coarsely chopped nuts

Preheat oven to 375°F (190°C). Combine flour, baking soda and salt; set aside. In a large mixer bowl, combine butter or margarine, granulated and brown sugars and vanilla. Beat until creamy. Beat in eggs. Add flour mixture; blend. Stir in chocolate morsels and nuts. Drop by rounded teaspoonfuls onto ungreased cookie sheets. Bake 8 to 10 minutes. Makes one-hundred 2-inch cookies.

Variation
Substitute whole-wheat flour for all or half the flour.

This recipe used by permission of the Nestlé Company.

Orange-Oatmeal Chippers

Outstanding orange flavor blends delicately with chocolate.

1/2 cup shortening
1 cup light brown sugar, lightly packed
1 egg
1 teaspoon grated orange peel
1 tablespoon orange juice
1/2 cup flour

1/4 teaspoon baking soda
1-1/2 cups uncooked quick-cooking
   rolled oats
1 (6-oz.) pkg. semisweet chocolate pieces
   (1 cup)
1/2 cup chopped walnuts

Grease cookie sheets; set aside. Preheat oven to 375°F (190°C). In a large mixer bowl, cream shortening and brown sugar. Beat in egg, orange peel and juice. Add flour and baking soda. Beat until smooth. Stir in oats, chocolate pieces and walnuts. Drop from a teaspoon onto prepared cookie sheets. Bake 10 to 12 minutes or until light brown. Makes 36 to 48 cookies.

Banana-Granola Cookies

Mashed bananas and molasses make a tasty, moist cookie.

1/3 cup shortening
1/2 cup light brown sugar, lightly packed
1/4 cup molasses
1 egg
1-1/3 cups mashed ripe bananas
   (3 to 4 bananas)
1/2 cup nonfat dry milk powder

1-1/4 cups flour
1 teaspoon baking powder
1/2 teaspoon baking soda
1/4 teaspoon salt
1/8 teaspoon ground ginger
2 cups granola cereal
1 cup semisweet chocolate pieces

Grease cookie sheets; set aside. Preheat oven to 350°F (175°C). In a large mixer bowl, cream shortening and brown sugar. Beat in molasses and egg. Stir in mashed bananas and dry milk. Combine flour, baking powder, baking soda, salt, and ginger. Blend into creamed mixture. Stir in granola and chocolate pieces. Drop from a teaspoon onto prepared cookie sheets. Bake 10 to 12 minutes. Cool on wire racks. Makes about 48 cookies.

Double-Chocolate Cookies

Chocolate twice-over satisfies the most persistent craving!

1/2 cup butter or margarine, room temperature	2 cups flour
1 cup sugar	1/2 cup unsweetened cocoa powder
1 egg	1/2 teaspoon baking soda
1 cup dairy sour cream	1/2 teaspoon salt
1 teaspoon vanilla extract	1/2 cup semisweet chocolate pieces

Grease cookie sheets; set aside. Preheat oven to 375°F (190°C). In a large mixer bowl, beat butter or margarine and sugar until fluffy. Beat in egg, then sour cream and vanilla. Combine flour, cocoa, baking soda and salt. Gradually beat into creamed mixture. Stir in chocolate pieces. Drop from a teaspoon onto prepared cookie sheets. Bake 8 to 10 minutes. Cool slightly before placing on wire racks. Makes about 60 cookies.

Crinkles

The tops resemble tortoise shell.

2 oz. unsweetened chocolate	2 teaspoons baking powder
1/2 cup shortening	1/2 teaspoon salt
1-2/3 cups sugar	1/3 cup milk
2 teaspoons vanilla extract	1/2 cup chopped walnuts
2 eggs	Sifted powdered sugar
2 cups flour	

Melt chocolate; set aside to cool. In a large mixer bowl, thoroughly cream shortening, sugar and vanilla. Beat in eggs, then melted chocolate. Combine flour, baking powder and salt. Add alternately with milk to chocolate mixture. Beat until blended. Stir in walnuts. Chill several hours. When ready to bake, preheat oven to 350°F (175°C). Grease cookie sheets. Form dough into 1-inch balls. Roll in sifted powdered sugar. Place on prepared cookie sheets 2 to 3 inches apart. Bake 15 minutes. Cool slightly before placing on wire racks. Makes about 48 cookies.

Unless indicated in the recipe, wait until bar cookies are cool before frosting.

Sour Cream Cookies

Delicate and moist—another accomplishment to add to your collection.

2 oz. unsweetened chocolate
2/3 cup butter or margarine,
  room temperature
1-1/3 cups sugar
1 teaspoon vanilla extract
1 egg

1/2 cup dairy sour cream
1-3/4 cups flour
1/2 teaspoon baking powder
1/2 teaspoon baking soda
1/2 teaspoon salt
1/2 cup chopped nuts

Grease cookie sheets; set aside. Melt chocolate; set aside. Preheat oven to 425°F (220°C). In a large mixer bowl, cream butter or margarine. Gradually beat in sugar, creaming well. Add vanilla and egg, beating until fluffy. Stir in melted chocolate, then sour cream. Add flour, baking powder, baking soda and salt. Stir until well-mixed. Stir in nuts. Drop by heaping teaspoonfuls onto prepared cookie sheets. Bake about 8 minutes. Cool slightly before placing on wire racks. Makes about 48 cookies.

Banana Oatmeal Drops

Chocolate, banana and nutmeg in an old-fashioned cookie.

3/4 cup butter or margarine,
  room temperature
1 cup light brown sugar, lightly packed
1 egg
1 cup mashed ripe banana (2 large)
1-1/2 cups flour
1/2 teaspoon salt

1/2 teaspoon baking soda
1/2 teaspoon nutmeg
1-1/2 cups uncooked quick-cooking
  rolled oats
1 (6 oz.) pkg. semisweet chocolate pieces
  (1 cup)

Preheat oven to 400°F (205°C). In a large mixer bowl, beat butter or margarine, brown sugar and egg until light and fluffy. Beat in bananas. Combine flour, salt, baking soda and nutmeg. Gradually beat into egg mixture. Stir in oats and chocolate pieces. Drop from a teaspoon onto ungreased cookie sheets 2 inches apart. Bake 12 to 15 minutes or until golden brown. Cool on wire racks. Makes 75 to 80 cookies.

Chocolate Macaroons

Chewy consistency and superb flavor.

6 oz. semisweet chocolate pieces
3 egg whites
1/4 teaspoon salt

1 cup sugar
1/2 cup ground blanched almonds
1/2 teaspoon vanilla extract

Melt chocolate pieces; set aside to cool. Grease cookie sheets; set aside. Preheat oven to 350°F (175°C). Beat egg whites and salt until stiff but not dry. Gradually beat in sugar until mixture is thick and glossy. Fold in almonds, vanilla and melted chocolate. Drop from a teaspoon onto cookie sheets. Bake 15 minutes. Cool on wire racks. Makes 36 to 40 cookies.

Marshmallow Sandwich Cookies

How about a dessert sandwich?

2 cups flour
1 teaspoon baking soda
1/4 teaspoon salt
1/4 cup unsweetened cocoa powder
1 cup granulated sugar
1 egg

1/3 cup cooking oil
1 teaspoon vanilla extract
3/4 cup milk
1/2 cup butter or margarine
1 cup powdered sugar
1/4 cup marshmallow creme

Grease cookie sheets; set aside. Preheat oven to 350°F (175°C). In a large mixer bowl, combine flour, baking soda, salt, cocoa and granulated sugar. Make a well in center of mixture; add egg, oil, vanilla and milk. Beat until smooth. Drop by rounded tablespoonfuls onto prepared cookie sheets about 3 inches apart. Bake 10 to 12 minutes. Cool on wire rack. In a small mixer bowl, combine butter or margarine, powdered sugar and marshmallow creme. Beat until smooth. Spread the cream filling on half the cooled cookies; top with remaining cookies. Makes about 14 cookies.

Pecan Rounds   *Photo on page 47.*

An impressive addition to a cookie tray.

2 oz. unsweetened chocolate
1 cup butter or margarine, room temperature
3/4 cup sugar
1 teaspoon vanilla extract
2 cups flour
1/4 teaspoon baking powder

1/4 teaspoon baking soda
1/4 cup finely chopped pecans
1/4 cup sugar
1/2 teaspoon cinnamon
Pecan halves for garnish

Melt chocolate; set aside to cool. Preheat oven to 350°F (175°C). In a large bowl, cream butter or margarine and 3/4 cup sugar. Stir in vanilla and melted chocolate. Combine flour, baking powder and baking soda. Stir into chocolate mixture. Add chopped pecans. Form into 1-inch balls. If dough is too soft to handle, refrigerate for a few minutes. Mix 1/4 cup sugar and the cinnamon. Roll balls in mixture. Press a pecan half onto top of each ball. Bake on ungreased cookie sheets 12 to 15 minutes or until firm. Makes about 55 cookies.

When dropping cookie dough from a teaspoon onto a cookie sheet, use the back of another teaspoon to push the dough off the spoon.

Coconut Chews

Meringue-type cookie with a chewy center.

4 egg whites
2 cups powdered sugar
2 cups finely crushed vanilla wafer crumbs
   (about 60 wafers)

2 tablespoons unsweetened cocoa powder
1/2 teaspoon cinnamon
1/2 cup flaked coconut

Grease cookie sheets; set aside. Preheat oven to 325°F (165°C). In a large mixer bowl, beat egg whites until soft peaks form. Gradually add powdered sugar, beating until stiff peaks form. Combine wafer crumbs, cocoa and cinnamon. Fold into egg white mixture. Fold in coconut. Drop from a teaspoon onto prepared cookie sheets 2 inches apart. Bake 20 minutes. Cool on wire racks. Makes 45 to 50 cookies.

Pretzel Cookies

Almond cookies in a new surprise shape.

1 cup butter or margarine, room temperature
1 cup sugar
3 egg yolks
1 cup ground unblanched almonds

1/4 teaspoon almond extract
1 teaspoon grated lemon peel
2-1/4 cups flour
Cookie Glaze, see below

Cookie Glaze:
1 (12-oz.) pkg. semisweet chocolate pieces
   (2 cups)
1/4 cup light corn syrup

2/3 cup milk
1 tablespoon butter or margarine

In a large mixer bowl, beat butter or margarine and sugar until fluffy. Add egg yolks 1 at a time, beating well after each addition. Add almonds, almond extract and lemon peel. Gradually add flour, mixing until dough is smooth. Cover and refrigerate 2 hours. Grease cookie sheets; set aside. Preheat oven to 350°F (175°C). Form dough into balls using about 1 tablespoon dough for each. On a lightly floured board using palms of hands, form each ball into a 10-inch-long roll. Twist into a pretzel shape. Place on prepared cookie sheets about 2 inches apart. Bake 10 to 12 minutes or until light brown. Cool on wire rack over wax paper or aluminum foil. Prepare Cookie Glaze. Carefully spoon glaze over warm cookies. Cool. Makes about 40 cookies.

Cookie Glaze:
While cookies are baking, combine chocolate pieces, corn syrup, milk and butter or margarine in a small saucepan. Stir constantly over low heat until chocolate melts.

Pinwheels

Fascinating flavor-color contrast!

1/2 cup butter or margarine, room temperature	1 teaspoon vanilla extract
3/4 cup sugar	1-1/2 cups flour
1 egg	1/4 teaspoon salt
	2 tablespoons unsweetened cocoa powder

In a large mixer bowl, cream butter or margarine, sugar and egg until light and fluffy. Stir in vanilla. Add flour and salt; mix until blended. Divide dough in half. Add cocoa to one half. Cover and refrigerate both halves several hours or until firm. On floured wax paper, roll each half of dough to a 16" x 6" rectangle. Invert white dough on chocolate dough; peel wax paper off white dough. Tightly roll up doughs together, peeling wax paper off chocolate dough as you roll. Cover rolls and refrigerate several hours or overnight. Preheat oven to 400°F (205°C). Slice roll 1/4 inch thick. If dough becomes soft while slicing, refrigerate briefly. Bake on ungreased cookie sheet 5 to 7 minutes or until lightly browned. Cool on wire rack. Makes 60 to 65 cookies.

Spritz Cookies   *Photo on page 47.*

A cookie press is available in most housewares departments.

1/4 cup boiling water	1 egg yolk
6 tablespoons unsweetened cocoa powder	2 cups flour
1 cup butter, room temperature	1/2 teaspoon baking powder
1 teaspoon vanilla extract	1/4 teaspoon salt
1/2 cup sugar	

In a small bowl, thoroughly mix boiling water and cocoa; set aside to cool. Preheat oven to 350°F (175°C). In a large mixer bowl, cream butter and vanilla. Add sugar gradually, beating until light and fluffy. Add egg yolk; beat thoroughly. Stir in cocoa mixture. Combine flour, baking powder and salt. Add to creamed mixture 1/4 at a time, mixing until blended after each addition. Put dough through a cookie press onto an ungreased cookie sheet. Bake 12 minutes. Cool on wire racks. Makes about 60 to 70 cookies.

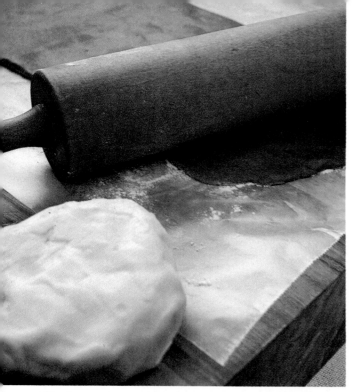

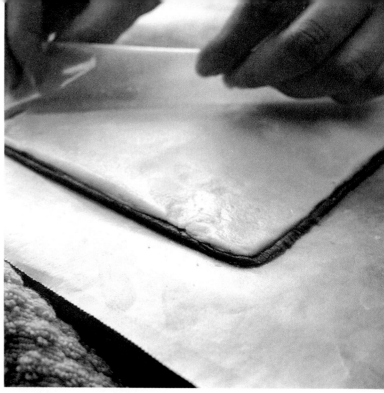

1/To form a two-toned pinwheel cookie, you'll need equal amounts of white or plain and chocolate dough. Refrigerate both doughs several hours for easier handling. Then on a small piece of wax paper, roll out each dough to a 16'' x 6'' rectangle.

2/Working as quickly as possible, invert the plain dough rectangle over the chocolate rectangle. Carefully peel off the wax paper from plain dough.

How To Make Pinwheels

3/With both hands, tightly roll up doughs together. Peel wax paper off the chocolate dough as you roll. Cover and chill several hours before slicing.

4/With a sharp knife, slice chilled dough crosswise about 1/4 inch thick. If dough begins to soften, refrigerate. When dough is firm again, continue slicing.

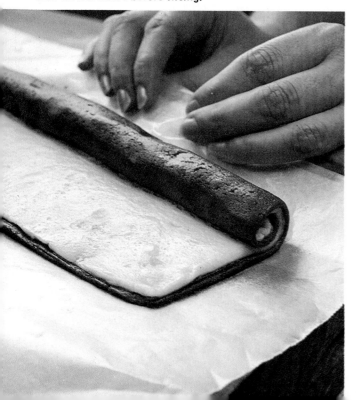

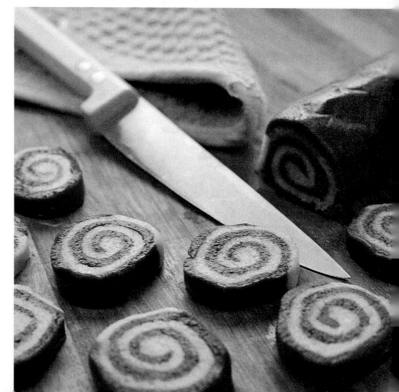

Kissing Cookies

Put a lot of love in your cookies with chocolate kisses.

1/2 cup butter or margarine, room temperature
3/4 cup creamy peanut butter
1/3 cup granulated sugar
1/3 cup light brown sugar, lightly packed
1 egg
2 tablespoons milk
1 teaspoon vanilla extract

1-1/2 cups flour
1 teaspoon baking soda
1/2 teaspoon salt
1/2 cup granulated sugar
1 (9-oz.) pkg. milk chocolate candy kisses, unwrapped

Preheat oven to 375°F (190°C). In a large mixer bowl, cream butter or margarine and peanut butter. Gradually beat in 1/3 cup granulated sugar and the brown sugar until light and fluffy. Add egg, milk and vanilla; mix well. Combine flour, baking soda and salt. Gradually blend into creamed mixture. Shape dough into 1-inch balls. Roll in 1/2 cup granulated sugar. Place on ungreased cookie sheet. Bake 10 to 12 minutes or until cracked and light brown. Remove from oven and immediately press a chocolate kiss firmly into center of each cookie. Carefully remove from cookie sheet. Cool on wire racks until chocolate is set, about 2 hours. Makes 48 to 50 cookies.

Acorn Cookies   *Photo on page 47.*

Eye appealing and palate pleasing!

1 cup butter, room temperature
3/4 cup light brown sugar, lightly packed
1 teaspoon vanilla extract
2-3/4 cups flour

1/2 teaspoon baking powder
1 (6-oz.) pkg. semisweet chocolate pieces
    (1 cup)
1/2 cup finely chopped pecans

Preheat oven to 350°F (175°C). In a medium mixing bowl, cream butter, brown sugar and vanilla. Stir in flour and baking powder. Using a rounded teaspoon of dough for each cookie, shape into balls. Pinch dough to a rounded point at one end to resemble an acorn. Place each on a cookie sheet either upright, rounded point up, or lying on one side. Bake about 15 minutes or until golden brown. Cool. Melt chocolate over hot but not boiling water. Dip large end of cooled cookie first into chocolate, then into chopped pecans. Makes about 48 cookies.

Candies

Making candy is fun! And it can be a family or party project with buttering the pan, measuring and preparing ingredients, cooking, beating and forming or cutting assigned to the participants. Usually they join in eagerly because the anticipation of the fruits of their labor suppresses all thoughts of candy making as work!

The economics of making your own candy has to be a distinct plus. Homemade candy is far less expensive than commercial products. In most cases, candy making is not a tedious and time-consuming process. At our house, a spur-of-the-moment craving for fudge often nudges us into the kitchen for a short candy-making session.

In making candy, the most critical phase is judging when to stop the cooking process. This is difficult to determine by cooking time, because no two stoves cook at exactly the same heat intensity on the identical heat settings. That's why it's best to rely on thermometer readings, the Cold Water Test below, or on both methods.

To test the accuracy of your candy thermometer, place it in a pan of warm water. Gradually bring the water to a boil and boil for 10 minutes. The thermometer should read 212°F (100°C). If it doesn't, add or subtract the number of degrees necessary for accuracy in cooking.

Cold Water Test		
Stage	**Temperature (at sea level)**	**When a small amount of syrup is dropped into a cup of cold water:**
Soft-ball	234° to 240°F 112° to 116°C	Syrup doesn't disintegrate but forms a recognizable soft ball that flattens on your finger when removed from water.
Firm-ball	244° to 248°F 118° to 120°C	Syrup holds ball shape when removed from water and flattens easily with slight finger pressure.
Hard-ball	250° to 266°F 121° to 130°C	Syrup holds ball shape when removed from water, shows slight resistence to finger pressure and is pliable.
Soft-crack	270° to 290°F 132° to 143°C	Syrup forms firm but not brittle threads.
Hard-crack	300° to 310°F 149° to 154°C	Syrup forms hard and brittle threads.

Creamy Rich Fudge

Exceptionally creamy fudge with strong chocolate flavor.

4 oz. unsweetened chocolate
1-1/4 cups milk
3 cups sugar
2 tablespoons light corn syrup

1/8 teaspoon salt
1/4 cup butter or margarine
1 teaspoon vanilla extract
1/2 cup chopped nuts

Lightly butter an 8-inch square pan; set aside. In a 3-quart saucepan, constantly stir chocolate and milk over low heat until chocolate melts. Stir in sugar, corn syrup and salt. Cook, stirring occasionally, until mixture reaches soft-ball stage or 236°F (113°C) on a candy thermometer. Remove from heat. Add butter or margarine. Cool at room temperature without stirring until temperature drops to 120°F (48°C) or bottom of pan feels warm, about 1 hour. Add vanilla; beat until candy loses its gloss and starts to thicken. Quickly stir in nuts. Pour into prepared pan. Cool until firm. Cut into squares. Makes about 36 pieces.

Peanut Butter Fudge

Our favorite—rich, creamy and delightfully peanutty!

4 cups sugar
1 teaspoon salt
1/2 cup unsweetened cocoa powder
1-1/3 cups milk

1/4 cup butter or margarine
2 teaspoons vanilla extract
3/4 cup peanut butter

Butter an 11" x 7-1/2" pan; set aside. In a 3-quart saucepan, combine sugar, salt and cocoa. Add milk; stir until blended. Cook over medium-low heat, stirring occasionally, until sugar just dissolves. Add butter or margarine. Continue cooking without stirring until mixture reaches soft-ball stage or 238°F (114°C) on a candy thermometer. Remove from heat. Cool at room temperature without stirring until bottom of pan is warm, about 120°F (48°C). Add vanilla and peanut butter. Beat until candy loses its gloss and begins to thicken. Pour into prepared pan. Cool until firm. Cut into squares. Makes 30 to 35 pieces.

Peanut Butter Chip Fudge

Peanut butter pieces partially melted in milk chocolate fudge create a swirled effect.

2 cups granulated sugar
1 cup light brown sugar, lightly packed
1 cup milk chocolate pieces
1 cup milk

2 tablespoons light corn syrup
2 tablespoons butter or margarine
1 teaspoon vanilla extract
1 small pkg. peanut butter pieces (1 cup)

Lightly butter an 8-inch square pan; set aside. In a 3-quart pan, combine granulated and brown sugars, chocolate pieces, milk and corn syrup. Bring to a boil, stirring until sugar dissolves. Cook over medium heat without stirring until mixture reaches the soft-ball stage, 236°F (113°C) on a candy thermometer. Remove from heat and add butter or margarine. Let cool without stirring until bottom of pan feels warm, about 120°F (48°C). Add vanilla; beat until candy thickens and begins to lose its gloss. Quickly stir in peanut butter pieces. Pour into prepared pan. Cool until firm. Cut into squares. Makes about 36 pieces.

Pronto Fudge

Marshmallow creme fudge is quick, easy and creamy with a medium chocolate flavor.

1/2 cup butter or margarine
3 cups sugar
1 (5.33-oz.) can evaporated milk, not diluted
1 (12-oz.) pkg. semisweet chocolate pieces
   (2 cups)

1 (7-oz.) jar marshmallow creme
1/2 cup chopped nuts
1 teaspoon vanilla extract

Lightly butter a 13" x 9" pan. In a heavy 2-1/2- or 3-quart saucepan, melt butter or margarine over low heat. Add sugar and evaporated milk. Stirring constantly, bring to a rolling boil over medium-low heat. Cook, stirring constantly, about 4 minutes or until mixture reaches 226°F (108°C) on a candy thermometer. Remove from heat. Add chocolate pieces. Beat with a spoon until melted. Stir in marshmallow creme, nuts and vanilla. Pour into prepared pan. Cool. Cut into squares. Makes about 60 pieces.

On humid days, cook candy syrup to 1 or 2 degrees higher than is called for in the recipe.

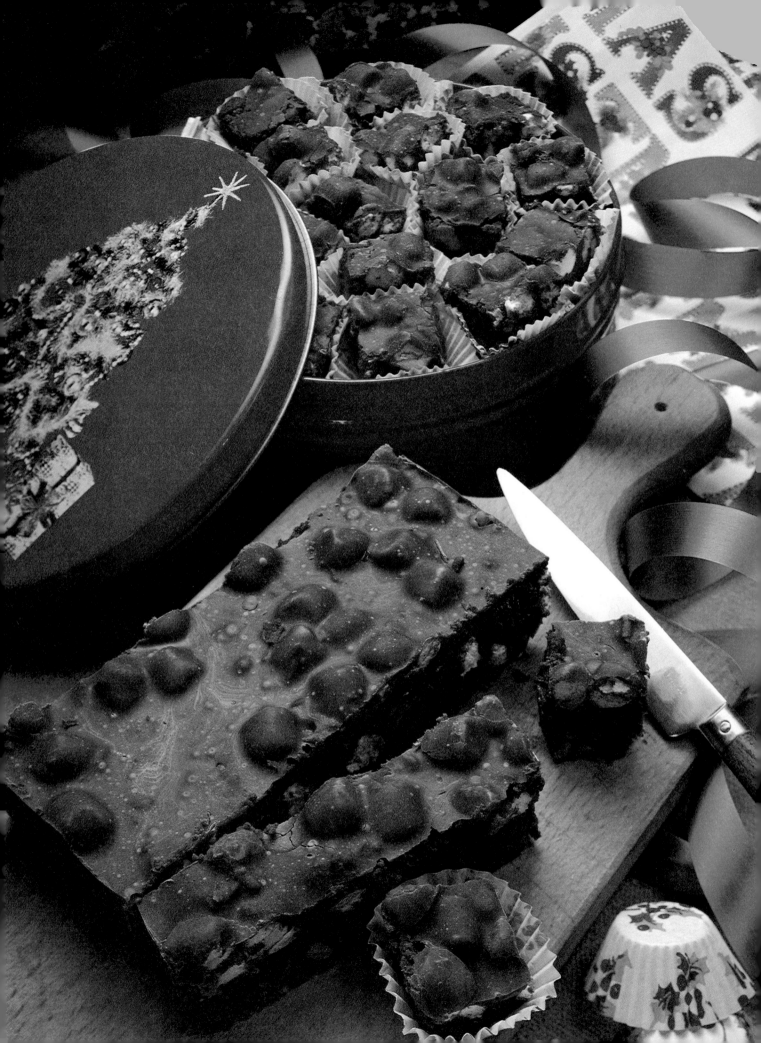

Holiday Rocky Road Fudge

Delicious fudge with all kinds of goodies mixed in.

3 cups sugar
3/4 cup unsweetened cocoa powder
1/2 cup light corn syrup
1 cup milk
1/4 cup butter or margarine

1 teaspoon vanilla extract
1/2 cup candied cherries, halved
1 cup miniature marshmallows
1/2 cup coarsely chopped nuts
1/2 cup flaked coconut

Lightly butter a 13" x 9" baking pan. In a 3-quart saucepan, combine sugar, cocoa, corn syrup and milk. Cook over moderate heat until sugar dissolves and mixture begins to boil. Continue cooking over medium-low heat, stirring occasionally, until mixture reaches soft-ball stage or 238°F (114°C) on a candy thermometer. Remove from heat. Add butter or margarine and vanilla, but do not stir. Cool to lukewarm. Beat until creamy. Stir in candied cherries, marshmallows, nuts and coconut. Pour into prepared pan. Cut into squares when cool. Makes about 50 squares.

No-Work Fudge

For those who like rich dark chocolate the easy way.

3 (6-oz.) pkgs. semisweet chocolate pieces
  (3 cups)
1 (14-oz.) can sweetened condensed milk

1 teaspoon vanilla extract
1/2 cup chopped walnuts

Butter an 8-inch square pan; set aside. In a 2-quart saucepan, melt chocolate pieces. Stir in condensed milk, vanilla and walnuts. Pour into prepared pan. Refrigerate about 2 hours or until firm. Cut into squares. Makes about 25 squares.

English Toffee

Crunchy toffee with chocolate-nut topping.

1 cup butter or margarine
1 cup sugar
2 tablespoons water
1 tablespoon light corn syrup

1/2 cup chopped walnuts
4 oz. sweet cooking chocolate
1/2 cup chopped walnuts

Lightly butter a cookie sheet; set aside. In a 2-quart saucepan, melt butter or margarine. Add sugar, water and corn syrup. Cook over low heat, stirring occasionally, until mixture reaches soft-crack stage or 290°F (143°C) on a candy thermometer. Remove from heat; quickly add 1/2 cup chopped walnuts. Spread about 1/4 inch thick on prepared cookie sheet. Cool thoroughly. Melt chocolate; cool slightly. Spread over cooled candy. Sprinkle with remaining 1/2 cup chopped walnuts. Refrigerate until firm. Break into small pieces. Makes 50 to 60 pieces.

Butter-Nut Crunch

Crunchy, yet melts in your mouth.

1 cup sugar
1/2 teaspoon salt
1/2 cup butter or margarine
1/4 cup water

1/2 cup chopped walnuts
1 (6-oz.) pkg. semisweet chocolate pieces
  (1 cup)
1/2 cup chopped walnuts

Butter a 15" x 10" cookie sheet; set aside. In a medium saucepan, combine sugar, salt, butter or margarine and water. Cook until mixture reaches soft-crack stage or 270°F (132°C) on a candy thermometer. Stir in 1/2 cup chopped walnuts. Pour onto prepared cookie sheet. If necessary, spread to about 1/4-inch thickness. Cool. Melt chocolate; spread over cooled candy. Sprinkle with remaining 1/2 cup chopped walnuts. When cool, break into irregular chunks. Makes 35 to 40 pieces.

Cocoa Pralines

Bet you can't eat just one!

2 cups light brown sugar, lightly packed
1 tablespoon unsweetened cocoa powder
1/8 teaspoon salt

2/3 cup evaporated milk, not diluted
2 tablespoons butter or margarine
1-1/2 cups whole pecans

Lightly butter a cookie sheet or large piece of aluminum foil. In a 2-quart saucepan, combine brown sugar, cocoa, salt, evaporated milk and butter or margarine. Stir constantly over low heat until sugar dissolves. Add pecans; stir constantly over medium heat, until mixture reaches soft-ball stage or 234°F (112°C) on a candy thermometer. Remove from heat; cool 5 minutes. Stir until mixture begins to thicken and coats pecans. Drop from a teaspoon onto prepared cookie sheet or foil, forming fairly flat round candies about 1-1/2- to 2-inches in diameter. If candy stiffens too much in saucepan, add a few drops of hot water. Makes about 30 pralines.

Quick French Creams

Easy to make, yet elegant!

8 oz. semisweet cooking chocolate
1 cup sifted powdered sugar
1 tablespoon milk

1 egg, well beaten
1/3 cup chocolate sprinkles

In top of a double boiler over hot but not boiling water, melt chocolate, stirring until smooth. Remove from water. Quickly stir in powdered sugar, milk and egg. Refrigerate until firm enough to shape. Form into 1-inch balls. Roll in chocolate sprinkles. Makes 35 to 40 balls.

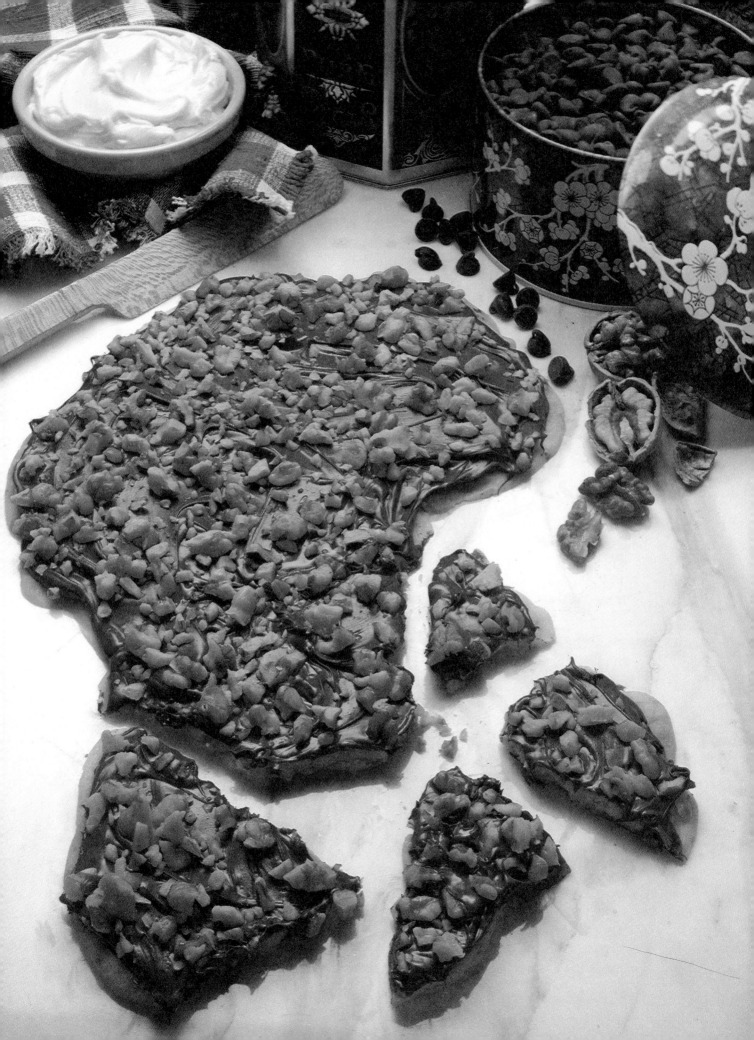

Two-Tone Mint Divinity

Each piece has a chocolate layer and a mint divinity layer.

1 oz. unsweetened chocolate
2-1/4 cups sugar
1/3 cup light corn syrup
1/3 cup water

2 egg whites
1/2 teaspoon vanilla extract
1/2 cup finely crushed peppermint stick candy

Melt chocolate; set aside. Lightly butter a 9" x 5" loaf pan. In a 2-quart saucepan, combine sugar, corn syrup and water. Bring to a boil, stirring until sugar dissolves. Boil over moderate heat without stirring until mixture reaches soft-ball stage or 236°F (113°C) on a candy thermometer. While mixture is boiling, beat egg whites in a large mixer bowl until stiff peaks form. Pour hot syrup very slowly over beaten egg whites, beating until mixture forms soft peaks. Pour half of mixture into another bowl. To remaining mixture add melted chocolate and vanilla. Spoon into prepared pan. Add peppermint candy to other half of mixture. Spoon over chocolate layer. Cool until set. Cut into squares. Makes about 32 squares.

Oasis Bonbons

So quick and easy, you'll think they're part of a mirage!

4 oz. sweet cooking chocolate
1 cup chunky peanut butter
1 cup powdered sugar

1/2 cup flaked coconut
1-1/2 cups chopped pitted dates
1 teaspoon grated orange peel

Line a cookie sheet with wax paper; set aside. Melt chocolate; set aside. In a medium bowl, combine peanut butter, powdered sugar, coconut, dates and orange peel. Shape into 1-inch balls. Dip top half of each ball into melted chocolate. Place on prepared cookie sheet with chocolate side up. Refrigerate until chocolate is set. Makes about 35 bonbons.

Bourbon Balls

A tantalizing blend of flavors.

1 (6-oz.) pkg. semisweet chocolate pieces
   (1 cup)
3 tablespoons light corn syrup
1/4 cup bourbon
1/2 cup sugar

1-1/4 cups vanilla wafer crumbs
   (about 38 wafers)
1 cup finely chopped walnuts
Powdered sugar

Melt chocolate. Stir in corn syrup, bourbon, sugar, vanilla wafer crumbs and walnuts. Using a heaping teaspoon of mixture for each piece, form into balls; roll in powdered sugar. Cover and refrigerate several hours. Makes about 36 balls.

Peanut Crisp

Peanuts, chocolate, marshmallow and cereal make a super afternoon snack.

1/2 cup butter or margarine
1 cup peanut butter
1 (11-1/2-oz.) pkg. milk chocolate pieces
   (about 2 cups)

1 (10-1/2-oz.) pkg. miniature marshmallows
4-1/4 cups crispy rice cereal
1 cup unsalted peanuts

Lightly butter a 13" x 9" baking pan; set aside. In a 3-quart saucepan, combine butter or margarine, peanut butter and half the chocolate pieces. Stir constantly over low heat until chocolate melts. Add marshmallows, stirring until melted. Stir in cereal and peanuts. Immediately pat mixture into prepared pan and sprinkle top with remaining chocolate pieces. Cover pan with cookie sheet or aluminum foil; let stand several minutes or until chocolate starts to melt. With a small spatula, smooth chocolate over top. Refrigerate until set. Cut into bars. Makes about 36 bars.

Pecan Penuche

Ever-popular penuche with a chocolate topping.

2 cups granulated sugar
2 cups light brown sugar, lightly packed
1/2 cup light cream
1/2 cup milk
3 tablespoons butter or margarine

1-1/2 teaspoons vanilla extract
1 cup coarsely chopped pecans
1/2 cup semisweet chocolate pieces
24 pecan halves

Butter an 8-inch square baking pan; set aside. Butter side of a 2-1/2- or 3-quart saucepan. Add granulated and brown sugars, cream, milk and butter or margarine. Cook over medium heat, stirring until sugar just dissolves and mixture boils. Boil without stirring until mixture reaches soft-ball stage or 236°F (113°C) on a candy thermometer. Remove from heat. Cool without stirring until bottom of pan is warm or to 120°F (50°C). Add vanilla. With electric mixer on high speed, beat until mixture thickens and begins to lose its gloss. Quickly stir in chopped pecans and pour into prepared pan, spreading evenly over bottom. While still warm but firm, cut into 24 pieces. Cool in pan. When candy in pan is cool, melt chocolate pieces. Spoon melted chocolate in a zig-zag pattern over top of candy. Place a pecan half on top of each piece of candy. Makes about 24 pieces.

A pan with a heavy bottom that holds about 4 times the volume of the ingredients minimizes the chances of scorching and boil-overs.

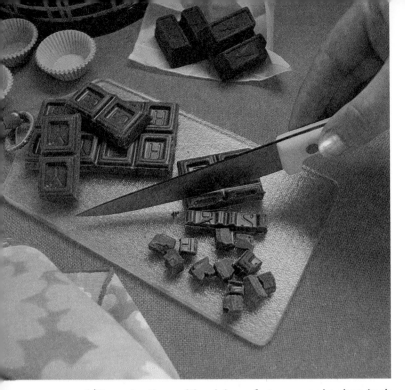

1/To make the melting job go faster, coarsely chop both kinds of chocolate before combining in the double boiler. Stir chocolate occasionally until it is melted and smooth.

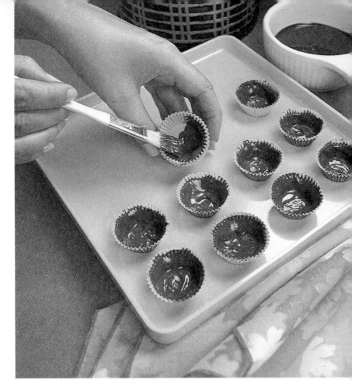

2/Small (1-1/2-inch) bonbon cups are just right for this job. With a clean, dry brush, carefully coat the side of each paper cup with the melted chocolate. It will be difficult to peel off the paper later if you go over the top edge. Chill the chocolate cups while you make the filling.

How To Make Mint Truffles

3/The filling is made of more chocolate with butter and eggs plus peppermint flavoring. When the mixture looks like chocolate-colored mayonnaise, it's time to fill the chilled cups. Spoon about one rounded teaspoonful of mixture into each cup.

4/After cups are filled, cover and refrigerate until serving time. They may be frozen for longer storage. While they are still cold, carefully peel off paper and serve.

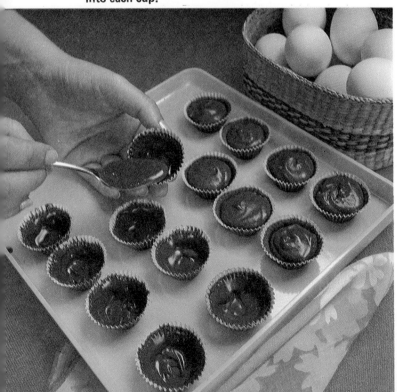

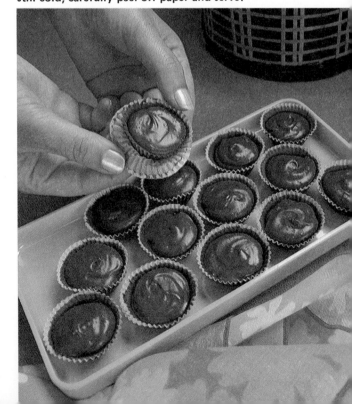

Mint Truffles

You'll need 36 (1-1/2-inch) fluted paper bonbon cups and a 1/2-inch brush.

2 oz. semisweet cooking chocolate
1 (8-oz.) milk chocolate candy bar,
   halved
4 oz. semisweet cooking chocolate

1/2 cup butter or margarine
3 eggs
1/8 teaspoon salt
1/2 teaspoon peppermint extract

Coarsely chop 2 ounces semisweet chocolate and 4 ounces milk chocolate (1/2 candy bar). Combine in top of a double boiler over hot but not boiling water. Stir occasionally until melted and smooth. Loosen top bon bon cup from stack, but leave in stack for greater stability while being coated. With a small, new dry paintbrush, coat the inside of the top cup evenly with melted chocolate, about 1/16" to 1/8" thick, bringing coating almost to top of cup but not over edge. Carefully remove coated cup from stack. Repeat until 36 cups are coated, stirring chocolate occasionally while you work. Refrigerate coated cups. Coarsely chop remaining half of candy bar and 4 ounces semisweet chocolate. In a small saucepan, melt butter or margarine until it bubbles and foams. Remove from heat. Add chopped chocolate; stir until melted and smooth. In a small mixer bowl, beat eggs and salt until foamy and lemon-colored. With electric mixer on high speed, very gradually add warm chocolate mixture. Mixture should be about the thickness of mayonnaise. Stir in peppermint extract. Drop by rounded teaspoonfuls into chocolate cups. Arrange single layer of filled cups in a 3/4-inch-deep pan or plastic container. Cover and refrigerate or freeze. To serve, peel off paper cups while candies are cold or frozen. Arrange in single layer on a serving plate. Makes about 36 pieces.

Quick Mint Patties

Party favorites and after-dinner nibblers.

3 tablespoons butter or margarine
3 tablespoons milk
1 (15.4-oz.) pkg. chocolate-fudge flavor
   frosting mix

1/2 teaspoon peppermint extract

Melt butter or margarine with milk in top of a double boiler. Stir in frosting mix. Cook over rapidly boiling water 5 minutes, stirring occasionally. Stir in peppermint. Drop from a teaspoon onto wax paper; swirl tops of candies with a spoon. If mixture becomes too thick, add a few drops of hot water. Cool candies until firm. Makes about 60 patties.

> *Do not stir boiling syrup unless instructed by the recipe. In many cases, especially with fudge, candy should not be stirred or beaten until it has cooled to a prescribed temperature.*

Mocha Pecan Logs

Dark chocolate with a touch of coffee.

1 cup light brown sugar, lightly packed
1/3 cup evaporated milk
2 tablespoons light corn syrup
1 (6-oz.) pkg. semisweet chocolate pieces
   (1 cup)

1 teaspoon instant coffee powder
1 teaspoon vanilla extract
1 cup chopped pecans

Grease a large cookie sheet; set aside. In a heavy medium saucepan, combine brown sugar, milk and corn syrup. Bring to a boil over medium heat, stirring constantly. Boil and stir 2 minutes. Remove from heat. Add chocolate pieces, coffee and vanilla, stirring until chocolate melts. With a wooden spoon, beat until thick and smooth. Stir in pecans. Spoon onto prepared cookie sheet in 2 equal parts. Shape each half into a 10-inch-long log. Wrap each log in wax paper. Refrigerate about 2 hours or until firm. Cut each log into 20 pieces. Makes 40 pieces.

Haystacks

The unique shape disguises their crunchy goodness.

1 (6-oz.) pkg. semisweet chocolate pieces
   (1 cup)
2 teaspoons cooking oil

1 (3-oz.) can chow mein noodles (2 cups)
2 cups miniature marshmallows

Line a cookie sheet with wax paper; set aside. Melt chocolate; stir in oil. In a large bowl, mix noodles and marshmallows. Pour melted chocolate mixture over noodles and marshmallows; stir with a fork. Drop by heaping teaspoonfuls onto wax paper. Refrigerate until firm. Makes about 30 pieces.

Peanut Butter Oatmeal Drops

Kids love these quick-to-make drops.

2 cups sugar
1/3 cup unsweetened cocoa powder
1/2 cup milk
1/4 cup butter

1/2 cup crunchy peanut butter
1 teaspoon vanilla extract
3 cups uncooked quick-cooking rolled oats

Line a cookie sheet with wax paper; set aside. In a medium saucepan, combine sugar and cocoa. Stir in milk and butter. Bring to a boil over medium heat, stirring constantly. Simmer about 2 minutes. Remove from heat. Stir in peanut butter and vanilla, then oats. Drop from a teaspoon onto wax paper. Cool until firm. Makes 38 to 46 pieces.

Dipping Your Own Chocolates

The Art Of Dipping Chocolate

Why would you want to spend your time dipping chocolates when you can buy beautifully made confections at the candy store? Sure it's fun, but for a beginner it can be extremely frustrating.

So you're determined to give it a try anyway. That's the first step to dipping chocolates successfully. You have to *want to learn how.*

If you've ever bitten into a beautiful but stale chocolate, you will appreciate your own chocolates. You will know the quality, flavor and freshness of the ingredients. Also, homemade chocolates are less expensive than comparable ones you can buy.

Although dipping chocolate is a practical and rewarding activity, it is a slow process and should not be hurried. Allow several hours for your project.

Like many hobbies, this may be difficult at first, but it is rewarding when you produce something beautiful. Dipping chocolates is a hobby that a family or a group can share. Think of the impressive array of candies you can make for Christmas!

There's no magic formula for beautiful, glossy chocolate-coated confections that can compare with the elegant commercial beauties. But keep trying—you'll be surprised!

Choosing Your Chocolate

Several kinds of chocolate can be used for dipping. The kind you choose should depend on taste, color and how easy it is to work with.

Dipping Chocolate—This is known by several names, including *dipping chocolate, chunk chocolate* and *chocolate bark.* Specially prepared for dipping, it is the easiest to use. This chocolate is sometimes available at candy stores, especially ones that make their own candy. Unfortunately, it is sold in quantities much larger than most of us need.

In some parts of the country during late fall, dipping chocolate is sold in chunks at supermarkets and variety stores. It comes in various quantities and a wide range of prices. If possible, buy a small amount of each, try them, and then purchase larger quantities of the kind you prefer. You'll probably have a choice of dark, milk or white chocolate. If the chocolate is prepackaged, directions for dipping are usually written on the label.

Milk chocolate and semisweet chocolate pieces—We found equal parts of milk chocolate pieces and semisweet chocolate pieces are the most practical combination for dipping. This blend provides a flavor that is a cross between dark and milk chocolate and has a very eye-appealing color.

Semisweet chocolate squares—This is the chocolate traditionally used by experienced candy dippers. Each 8-ounce box contains 8 individually wrapped 1-ounce squares. When used for dipping, these squares create a rich dark chocolate coating. This chocolate is more temperamental than the two above and is more difficult for a beginner to use.

Step-by-step directions for dipping chocolate begin on page 74.

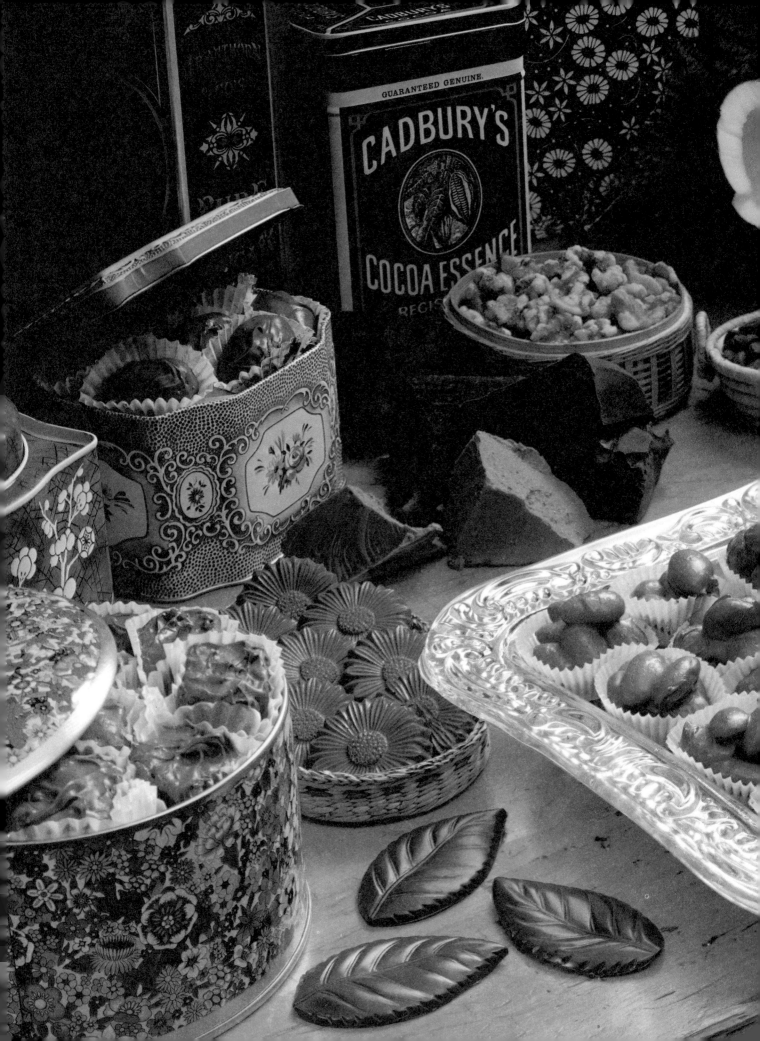

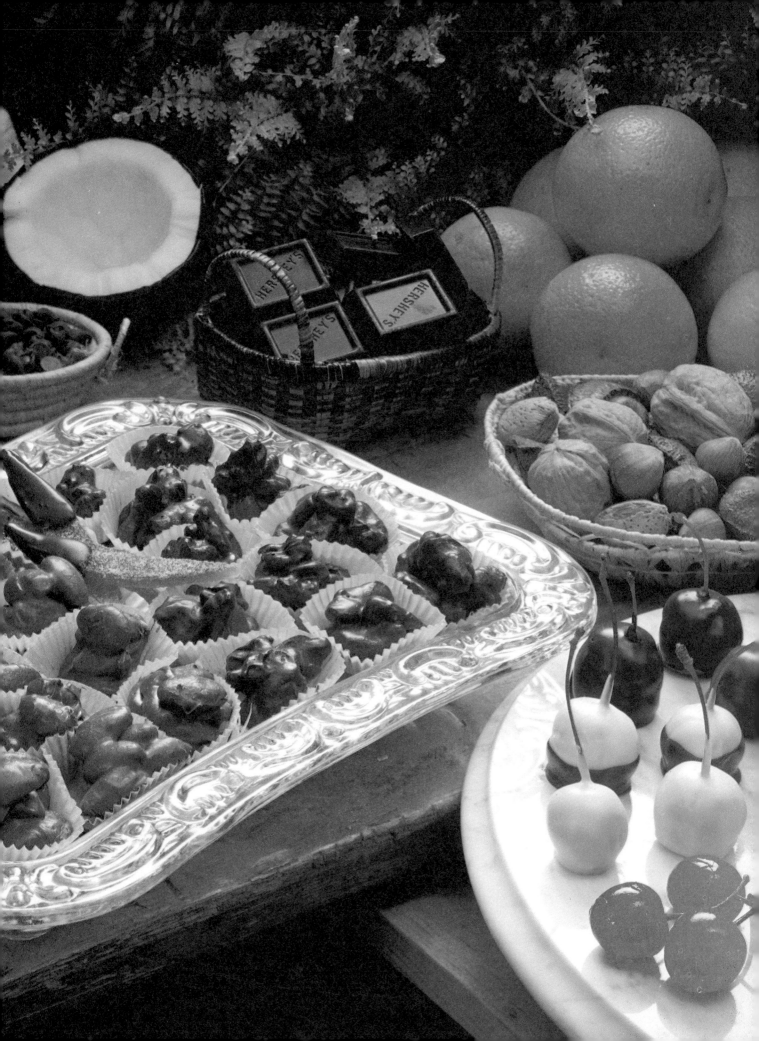

Dipping With Semisweet Chocolate Squares

1 (16-oz.) pkg. semisweet chocolate squares
70 to 80 centers, pages 77 to 79
Nuts or raisins, as desired

1. Unwrap chocolate squares and chop finely. Place in top of double boiler.

2. Pour almost boiling water about 2 inches deep into bottom of double boiler. Water should not touch the bottom of top part of double boiler.

3. Place the top of double boiler with chocolate over hot water. Do not place double boiler on heating unit.

4. Stir chocolate constantly until melted so it will melt evenly.

5. Insert thermometer in melted chocolate. Continue stirring vigorously until temperature reaches 130°F (54°C). Remove top of double boiler from hot water.

6. Pour hot water from bottom of double boiler. Replace with cold tap water. Place top of double boiler with melted chocolate over cold water. Stir and scrape side of pan with a spoon or spatula until temperature of chocolate is 83°F (28°C). If necessary, replace cold water in bottom of double boiler once or twice.

7. Maintain chocolate at 83°F (28°C), which is the recommended dipping temperature for semisweet chocolate squares. Replace water in bottom of double boiler with slightly warmer or cooler water as needed during the dipping.

8. Drop 1 center into chocolate. Stir with a fork. Slip fork under coated center and lift out quickly. Rap fork on edge of pan several times, then draw fork and center across rim of pan to remove excess chocolate.

9. Invert dipped center on wax paper or foil-covered wire rack. As the fork is removed, a thread of chocolate will fall across top of candy to form a design. Expert candy dippers form a different design for each flavor of candy to identify varieties.

10. Continue to stir melted chocolate as often as possible during dipping process. Work quickly and check the temperature of the chocolate frequently.

11. When there's very little chocolate left in pan, drop in small items such as nuts or raisins. Stir until well-coated. Pick up in clusters with a spoon and drop on wax paper or foil on wire rack.

12. Cool candies until set. Makes 70 to 80 pieces.

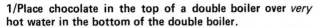

1/Place chocolate in the top of a double boiler over *very* hot water in the bottom of the double boiler.

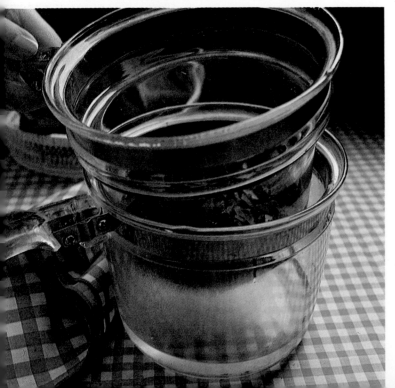

2/To check temperature, insert thermometer into chocolate and attach to side of pan.

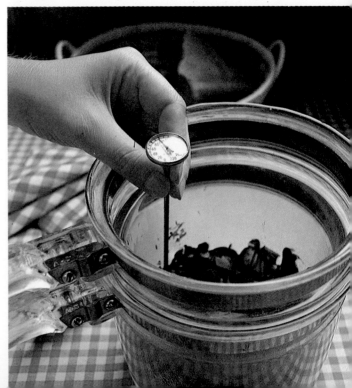

Dipping With Milk Chocolate And Semisweet Chocolate Pieces

1 (6-oz.) pkg. milk chocolate pieces (1 cup)
1 (6-oz.) pkg. semisweet chocolate pieces (1 cup)
50 to 60 centers, pages 77 to 79
Nuts or raisins, as desired

1. Place milk chocolate pieces and semisweet chocolate pieces into the top of a double boiler.
2. Pour almost boiling water about 2 inches deep into bottom of double boiler. The hot water should not touch the bottom of top part of double boiler.
3. Place the top of double boiler with chocolate over hot water. Do not place double boiler on heating unit.
4. Stir chocolate constantly until melted so it will melt evenly.
5. Insert thermometer in melted chocolate. Continue to stir vigorously until temperature reaches 108°F (42°C). Immediately remove top of double boiler from bottom pan of hot water.
6. Pour hot water from bottom of double boiler. Replace with cold tap water. Place top of double boiler with melted chocolate over cold water. Stir and scrape side of pan with a spoon or spatula until temperature is 80°F (27°C). If necessary, replace cold water in bottom of double boiler once or twice. Keep chocolate at 80°F (27°C) for 5 minutes, stirring vigorously. Remove from cold water.
7. Pour cold water from bottom of double boiler.

Replace with warm water, 90°F (32°C) to 95°F (35°C). Place top of double boiler with chocolate over warm water. Stir constantly until chocolate warms to 86°F (30°C). This is the recommended dipping temperature for the combination of milk chocolate pieces with semisweet pieces. Maintain this temperature throughout dipping. If necessary, replace water in bottom of double boiler with slightly warmer or cooler water.
8. Drop 1 center into chocolate. Stir well with a fork. Slip fork under coated center and lift out quickly. Rap fork on edge of pan several times, then draw fork and center across rim of pan to remove excess chocolate.
9. Invert dipped center on wax paper or foil-covered wire rack. As fork is removed, a thread of chocolate will fall across top of candy to form a design. Expert candy dippers form a different design for each flavor of candy to identify varieties.
10. Continue to stir melted chocolate as often as possible during dipping process. Work quickly and check the temperature of the chocolate frequently.
11. When there is very little chocolate left in the pan, drop in small items such as nuts or raisins. Stir until well-coated. Pick up in clusters with a spoon. Drop on wax paper or foil on wire rack.
12. Cool candies until set. Makes 50 to 60 pieces.

3/While melting chocolate and dipping candies, stir chocolate as much as possible to maintain an even temperature.

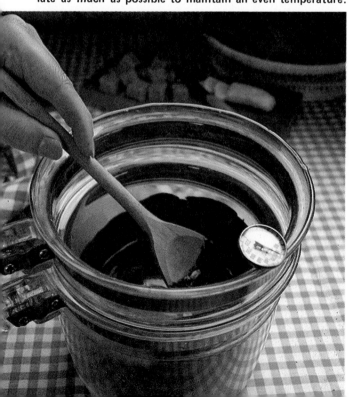

4/When chocolate reaches the correct dipping temperature, drop in a candy center. Lift out with a fork.

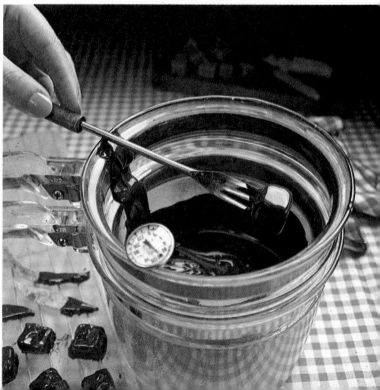

Getting Ready

☐ At least one day ahead, prepare the various flavors of fondant, creams, candied orange peel, caramels, nut fillings or fruit to be used as centers.

☐ If possible, choose a cool, clear day with low humidity for dipping. Moisture in the air can dull your chocolates. Temperatures in the room where you are dipping should be between 60° and 70°F (13° to 20°C).

☐ Do not work in an area where candies will be in a draft. If it's necessary to cool the room, open a window in an adjoining room or partially open a window where the draft will not blow on the candies.

☐ It is not necessary to dip candies at the heating units of your range. In fact, it is better to be away from the heat. Although you'll need almost boiling water to start melting chocolate, keep candies away from the hot oven or steam from a boiling pot or tea kettle.

☐ Assemble the equipment. You'll need:
- A double boiler or bowl that will fit in a pan without its bottom touching hot water.
- A spoon or rubber spatula for stirring.
- A kitchen or fondue fork for dipping candies.
- A thermometer with a range of at least from 80° to 130°F (27° to 54°C). Some candy thermometers or bi-therm thermometers have this range. You are most likely to find them in gourmet kitchen shops.
- A cooling rack covered with wax paper or aluminum foil.

☐ Have candy centers ready; place them near the dipping equipment. If you are dipping cherries, dip them into the fondant and let stand while melting chocolate. Form or cut other candy centers into desired shapes.

Now you are ready. The two following methods have been fully tested. Follow them carefully and they should give good results.

ON THE WAY TO SUCCESS

- Cut and shape candy centers before preparing chocolate. Flat, thin centers are harder to dip than rounded or cubed ones.
- Don't make the centers too large. Remember, chocolate coating adds to the size of the candies.
- The centers should be at room temperature when dipping.
- Make sure all your equipment and utensils are clean and dry.
- Less than 3/4 pound of melted chocolate is difficult to dip into. More than 2 pounds is hard to handle. Work with an amount in between.

- The ideal temperature for dipping varies with the kind of chocolate. Unless you are experienced in chocolate dipping, use the exact combination of chocolate and temperature we suggest. The temperature of the room as well as the temperature of the chocolate is important for successful dipping; see Getting Ready, above.
- Do not let any water fall into chocolate; it will cause the chocolate to *tighten* or stiffen and spoil the whole batch.
- Before moving dipped chocolates, cool until completely set. The chocolate should be firm.

Plain Fondant

Basic fondant for Cordial Cherries, page 79, or for chocolate dipped centers.

2 cups sugar
3/4 cup water
1 tablespoon light corn syrup

1/8 teaspoon salt
1 teaspoon vanilla extract

If you don't have a marble surface to work on, cool a 15" x 9" cookie sheet in the refrigerator. In a 2-quart saucepan, combine sugar, water, corn syrup and salt. Stir constantly over medium heat until sugar dissolves and mixture boils. Cover and cook over low heat for 3 minutes. Uncover. Insert candy thermometer in mixture. Continue cooking without stirring until mixture reaches 240°F (115°C) or soft-ball stage. Remove from heat. Pour onto clean and dry marble surface or chilled cookie sheet. Cool without stirring until center of fondant is lukewarm. With a spatula or wooden spoon, scrape fondant from edge toward center, turning occasionally, until creamy and stiff. When fondant loses its gloss and becomes crumbly, knead with your hands until smooth and soft. At first, kneading will seem impossible but the heat from your hands will soften the fondant. Add vanilla. Continue kneading until blended. Wrap in plastic wrap and refrigerate in a covered jar at least 24 hours. Makes 40 to 45 centers for dipping.

Cream Fondant

Rich creamy fondant in 2 delectable flavors for dipping into chocolate.

2 cups sugar
1/4 cup hot water
3/4 cup whipping cream
2 tablespoons light corn syrup
1 tablespoon butter
1/2 teaspoon vanilla extract

1/8 teaspoon peppermint extract
4 drops red food coloring
1/2 teaspoon grated orange peel
1/4 cup finely chopped coconut
4 drops orange food coloring

If you do not have a marble surface to work on, cool a 15" x 9" cookie sheet in the refrigerator. In a 2-quart saucepan, combine sugar, hot water, cream and corn syrup. Stir constantly over medium heat until mixture boils. Reduce heat to low. Cover and cook 3 minutes. Remove cover. Continue cooking without stirring until mixture reaches 240°F (115°C) on a candy thermometer or soft-ball stage. Remove from heat. Without scraping pan, immediately pour mixture onto clean and dry marble surface or chilled cookie sheet. Dot top with butter but do not stir. Cool until center is lukewarm. With a spatula or wooden spoon, scrape fondant from edge toward center, turning occasionally, until creamy and stiff. When mixture loses its gloss and becomes crumbly, knead with your hands until smooth and soft. As you begin, kneading will seem impossible, but the heat from your hands will soften the mixture. Add vanilla. Continue kneading until blended. Wrap in plastic wrap and refrigerate 24 hours in a covered jar. When ready to dip into chocolate, divide fondant in half. Knead peppermint extract and red food coloring into one half, then knead orange peel, coconut and orange-food coloring into the other half. Form each half into a roll 1 inch in diameter. Slice rolls 1/2 inch thick. Form some slices into cubes and ovals for variety in shapes. Place on wax paper. Cover and let stand several hours at room temperature before dipping into chocolate. Makes 45 to 50 centers for dipping.

Chocolate Marzipan

Chocolate-almond centers will blend subtly with a chocolate coating.

4 oz. almond paste
1 egg white

2 cups sifted powdered sugar
2 tablespoons unsweetened cocoa powder

In a small mixer bowl, with electric mixer on low speed, break almond paste into small pieces. Beat in egg white until smooth, several minutes. Beat in about half the powdered sugar. Turn out on a smooth surface. Knead in remaining powdered sugar and cocoa. Shape into 3/4-inch balls or ovals. Refrigerate in a covered bowl until ready to dip. Makes about 50 centers for dipping.

Peanut Butter Squares

Crunchy squares give a new shape and texture to dipped chocolate.

1/4 cup butter
1/3 cup chunky peanut butter
1/2 cup light corn syrup
1 tablespoon water

1 teaspoon vanilla extract
1 (1-lb.) box powdered sugar (4 cups)
1/3 cup instant nonfat dry milk powder

Butter an 8-inch square pan; set aside. In top of a double boiler over boiling water, combine butter and peanut butter. Stir until butter melts. Add corn syrup, water and vanilla. Mix well. Combine powdered sugar and dry milk. Gradually stir sugar mixture into peanut butter mixture. Heat over boiling water until smooth. Pour into prepared pan. Cool before cutting into squares. Makes 36 centers for dipping.

Butterscotch-Pecan Squares

You won't be able to resist nibbling these praline-flavored confections while dipping.

1 cup light brown sugar, lightly packed
1/4 cup butter
3 tablespoons milk

2 cups sifted powdered sugar
1/4 cup chopped pecans
1 teaspoon vanilla extract

Butter an 8-inch square pan; set aside. In a 2-quart saucepan, combine brown sugar, butter and milk. Bring to a boil, stirring constantly. Simmer 5 minutes. Remove from heat. Stir in powdered sugar, pecans and vanilla. Pour into prepared pan. Cool. When firm, cut into squares. Makes 45 to 50 centers for dipping.

When using fondant as centers for chocolate-dipped candies, add flavorings such as mint, orange, lemon and maple.

Brown Sugar Operas

Brown sugar squares make delicious centers for dipped chocolates.

1 cup granulated sugar
1 cup light brown sugar, lightly packed
1 tablespoon light corn syrup

3/4 cup sweetened condensed milk
1 cup whole milk
1/2 teaspoon vanilla extract

Butter an 8-inch square pan; set aside. In a heavy 2-quart saucepan, combine granulated and brown sugars. Stir in corn syrup, condensed milk and whole milk. Bring to a boil and cook, stirring constantly until mixture reaches 234°F (112°C) on a candy thermometer or soft-ball stage. Stir in vanilla. Cool to lukewarm. Beat until mixture is creamy, has thickened and is no longer glossy. Pour into prepared pan. Cool. Cut into squares. Makes 36 centers for dipping.

Cordial Cherries

A few days standing time gives the fondant and cherries a chance to create the delicious liquid layer.

1 (8-oz.) jar maraschino cherries with stems
1/2 recipe Plain Fondant

Chocolate for dipping, page 74 or 75

Drain cherry juice; place cherries on paper towels. Melt fondant in top of double boiler over hot water until it becomes a thick syrup. Place a sheet of wax paper on working surface. Dip drained cherries 1 at a time into fondant syrup, completely covering each cherry. Place on wax paper to cool. When syrup-covered cherries are completely cooled, prepare chocolate for dipping. Dip the bottom half of each cherry into chocolate. Return to wax paper and let harden. Line a tray or baking sheet with wax paper. When chocolate on cherries has cooled and hardened, dip again; this time completely coat each cherry with chocolate. Cool on prepared tray or baking sheet. Let stand in a cool dry place 2 or 3 days. Makes about 30 candies.

Tipped Candied Orange Peel

Prepare the orange peel 24 hours before dipping.

2 medium oranges
Water
1/2 cup light corn syrup
1 cup sugar

1 cup water
Sugar
Chocolate for dipping, page 74 or 75

With a knife, score peel of orange into 6 sections. Remove peel from oranges in scored sections. In a medium saucepan, cover peel with water. Heat to boiling. Boil 10 minutes. Drain. Repeat covering with water, boiling and draining 2 more times. After each cooking period, gently scrape off some of the soft white membrane with a spoon. Cut peel into strips about 1/4 inch wide. Combine corn syrup, 1 cup sugar and 1 cup water in a 2-quart saucepan. Stir constantly over medium heat until sugar dissolves. Add strips of orange peel. Bring to a boil. Simmer 45 minutes. Drain and cool. Roll strips in sugar. Arrange in a single layer on baking sheets. Let stand at room temperature about 24 hours before dipping. Picking up a few orange strips in your fingers, dip ends only into melted chocolate. Place on baking sheet to harden. Makes 45 to 50 pieces.

Custards, Puddings & Creams

The recipes in this group are based on delectable blends of chocolate with eggs and milk or cream. They range in variety and simplicity from plain Baked Cocoa Custard to elegant Charlotte Russe. Some are baked while others are either steamed or cooked in a saucepan.

When steaming a pudding, be sure to cover the mold. If it does not have a lid that clamps on, cover the mold with foil and tie it tightly with a string. Place the mold on a metal rack in a large kettle or steamer and pour water in the kettle around the mold. Cover the kettle so the heated water will steam the mold. Steam cooking is a slow process, so allow several hours for a steamed pudding.

Stirred puddings and custards, those cooked in a saucepan, are usually a custard mixture with different flavorings. The more elaborate ones have whipped cream, gelatin, nuts and liqueurs for a glamorous look and taste. For a smooth texture, keep the heat low and stir chocolate mixtures while they are cooking. Neither eggs nor chocolate cook well at high temperatures. If your custard mixture looks slightly grainy or if chocolate flecks remain, beat it with a wire whisk or rotary beater. Naturally, all dishes made with eggs or milk products should be kept in the refrigerator until serving time.

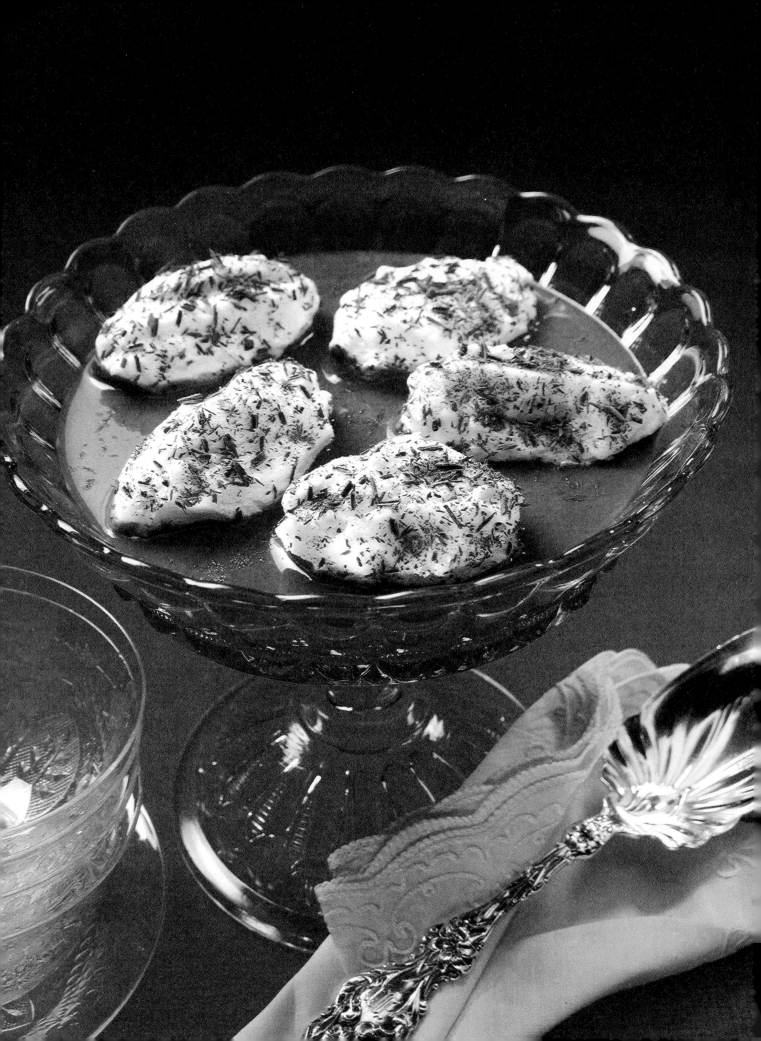

Floating Islands

Divine cloud-like meringues on heavenly chocolate custard.

3 egg whites	1/3 cup sugar
3/4 cup sugar	2 tablespoons unsweetened cocoa powder
2-1/2 cups milk	1/8 teaspoon nutmeg
3 egg yolks	Grated sweet chocolate, if desired

In a small mixer bowl, beat egg whites until foamy. Gradually beat in 3/4 cup sugar until meringue is stiff but not dry. In a large skillet over low heat, bring milk to a simmer. With a large spoon, scoop meringue into 5 egg-shaped puffs. Gently drop 1 at a time into hot milk. Cover and cook over very low heat 5 minutes. Lift out meringues with a slotted spoon. Drain on paper towels; chill. Remove milk from heat; set aside. In a small mixer bowl, beat egg yolks until thickened and lemon-colored. Gradually add 1/3 cup sugar. Beat in cocoa and nutmeg. Strain milk from skillet into egg yolk mixture. Mix until blended. Pour blended mixture into skillet. Stir constantly over low heat until mixture thickens slightly. Pour into a large shallow serving bowl. Chill. Just before serving, float meringues on top of chocolate custard. Sprinkle with grated sweet chocolate, if desired. Makes 5 servings.

Baked Cocoa Custard

For all custard fans!

3 eggs, slightly beaten	2 tablespoons unsweetened cocoa powder
2/3 cup sugar	2-1/2 cups milk
1 teaspoon vanilla extract	Nutmeg

Preheat oven to 350°F (175°C). In a medium bowl, combine eggs, sugar, vanilla and cocoa. Stir in milk. Pour into six 6-ounce custard cups. Sprinkle with nutmeg. Place cups in a 13" x 9" baking pan. Pour almost boiling water 1 inch deep into pan. Bake 45 minutes or until knife inserted into a custard comes out clean. Serve warm or cold. Makes 6 servings.

When cooling a custard mixture, place plastic wrap or wax paper directly on the surface of the custard to prevent a film from forming.

Chocolate Cream Pudding

Really great and easy to make.

1 cup sugar	2 egg yolks, slightly beaten
2 tablespoons cornstarch	2 tablespoons butter or margarine
1/4 teaspoon salt	1 teaspoon vanilla extract
2 cups milk	
2 oz. unsweetened chocolate, cut in small chunks	

In a medium saucepan, combine sugar, cornstarch and salt. Stir in milk and chocolate. Stir constantly over low heat until thickened and bubbly. Cook and stir 2 minutes more. Remove from heat. Stir a small amount of hot mixture into beaten egg yolks. Add egg yolk mixture to remaining hot mixture in saucepan. Cook and stir 2 minutes more. Remove from heat. Stir in butter or margarine and vanilla. Pour into dessert dishes. Chill. Makes 4 to 6 servings.

Cocoa Nut Pudding

Old-fashioned chocolate pudding like Grandma used to make.

2/3 cup sugar	2 egg yolks, slightly beaten
2 tablespoons cornstarch	1 tablespoon butter
2 tablespoons unsweetened cocoa powder	1 teaspoon vanilla extract
1/8 teaspoon salt	1/4 cup chopped walnuts
2 cups milk	

In a medium saucepan, combine sugar, cornstarch, cocoa and salt. Stir in milk and egg yolks. Cook over medium heat until mixture comes to a boil. Simmer 1 minute longer. Remove from heat. Stir in butter, vanilla and walnuts. Pour into a serving bowl. Cover and cool. Makes 4 or 5 servings.

Tropical Tapioca

An old favorite with an exotic flair.

3 tablespoons uncooked quick-cooking tapioca	2 cups milk
1/2 cup sugar	2 tablespoons sweetened instant cocoa mix
1/4 teaspoon salt	1/4 cup flaked coconut
2 eggs, slightly beaten	1 (11-oz.) can mandarin oranges, drained

In a heavy medium saucepan, combine tapioca, sugar, salt, eggs, milk and cocoa mix. Stir constantly over low heat until mixture boils. Cool slightly. Fold in coconut and half of mandarin oranges. Pour into a serving bowl or individual sherbet glasses. Garnish with remaining oranges. Chill. Makes 5 to 6 servings.

Steamed Fudge Pudding

Second helpings are the rule rather than the exception!

3 oz. unsweetened chocolate
2 tablespoons butter or margarine,
  room temperature
1/2 cup sugar
2 eggs
2 teaspoons baking powder

1/4 teaspoon salt
1 teaspoon vanilla extract
2 cups flour
1 cup milk
1/2 cup chopped walnuts
Sugar-Cream Sauce, see below

Sugar-Cream Sauce:
1/2 cup butter or margarine
1 cup sugar

1/2 cup light cream
1/2 teaspoon vanilla extract

Melt chocolate; set aside. Grease a 1-1/2 quart mold; set aside. In a medium mixing bowl, cream butter or margarine and sugar until light and fluffy. Beat in eggs. Stir in baking powder, salt and vanilla. Beat in flour alternately with milk. Add melted chocolate and walnuts. Stir until blended. Pour into prepared mold. Cover with aluminum foil and press overhanging foil edges against outside of mold. Loop a large rubber band over foil and around top of mold to seal, or tie foil securely with string. Place mold on a rack in a large pot. Pour enough water in pot to reach halfway up the mold. Cover pot. Bring to a boil; simmer 1-1/2 hours or until skewer inserted in pudding comes out clean. Remove mold from pot. Cool on wire rack 10 minutes. Prepare Sugar-Cream Sauce. Unmold pudding. Spoon sauce over warm pudding. Makes 8 to 10 servings.

Sugar-Cream Sauce:
Combine butter or margarine, sugar, cream and vanilla in a medium saucepan. Heat to boiling.

Steamed Date Pudding

An inviting dessert for a cold evening.

1/3 cup butter or margarine,
  room temperature
1 cup light brown sugar, lightly packed
2 eggs
2 tablespoons unsweetened cocoa powder
1 teaspoon baking soda
1-1/2 cups flour

1 cup water
1 (6-oz.) pkg. semisweet chocolate pieces
  (1 cup)
1 cup finely chopped pitted dates
1/2 cup chopped walnuts
1 teaspoon orange peel

Grease and flour a 1-1/2 quart mold; set aside. In a large mixer bowl, cream butter or margarine and brown sugar. Beat in eggs, then cocoa and baking soda. Add flour alternately with water, beating after each addition. With a spoon, stir in chocolate pieces, dates, walnuts and orange peel. Pour into prepared mold. Cover with aluminum foil and press overhanging foil edges against outside of mold. Loop a large rubber band over foil and around top of mold to seal, or tie foil securely with string. Place mold on a rack in a large kettle. Pour enough boiling water in kettle to reach halfway up the mold. Cover kettle. Simmer about 2 hours or until skewer inserted in pudding comes out clean. Remove mold from kettle. Let stand 15 minutes. Loosen edges with a knife and invert on a serving platter. Serve warm. Makes 8 to 10 servings.

Fudge-Top Pudding

Light delicate cake on top with rich fudge sauce on the bottom.

1 cup flour	2 tablespoons cooking oil
3/4 cup granulated sugar	1/2 cup chopped walnuts
2 tablespoons unsweetened cocoa powder	1 cup light brown sugar, lightly packed
2 teaspoons baking powder	1/4 cup unsweetened cocoa powder
1/4 teaspoon salt	1-3/4 cups hot water
1/2 cup milk	Whipped cream, if desired

Preheat oven to 350°F (175°C). In a medium bowl, combine flour, granulated sugar, 2 tablespoons cocoa, baking powder and salt. Add milk and oil; stir until smooth. Stir in walnuts. Pour into an ungreased 9-inch square pan. Combine brown sugar and 1/4 cup cocoa. Sprinkle over batter. Pour hot water over all, but *do not stir*. Bake 40 to 45 minutes. Pudding will be done when topping begins to leave the sides of pan although the center may not appear firm. Serve warm. Spoon the cake-like top upside down into dessert dishes. Spoon sauce from bottom of pan over each serving. Top with whipped cream, if desired. Makes 8 or 9 servings.

Royal Velvet Mousse

The smoothest and richest mousse!

3 egg yolks, room temperature	1/2 cup butter
3/4 cup sugar	2 tablespoons coffee liqueur
2 tablespoons water	3 egg whites, room temperature
1 oz. unsweetened chocolate	1/4 teaspoon cream of tartar
2 oz. semisweet chocolate	1/2 cup whipping cream

In a medium mixing bowl, beat egg yolks until thickened and lemon-colored or about 4 minutes. Heat sugar and water in a small saucepan until mixture begins to boil. Gradually pour over egg yolks, beating constantly. Heat unsweetened and semisweet chocolates and butter until chocolate melts. Add liqueur; set aside. Place bowl with egg yolk mixture over a pan of almost boiling water. Beat egg yolk mixture 5 minutes or until doubled in volume. Remove from hot water. Beat another 5 minutes. Fold chocolate mixture into egg yolks. In a small bowl, beat egg whites with cream of tartar until stiff but not dry. Fold beaten egg whites into chocolate mixture. Beat whipped cream in a small bowl. Fold into chocolate mixture. Spoon into a large serving bowl or dessert dishes. Refrigerate or freeze. If frozen, remove from freezer a few minutes before serving. Makes 6 to 8 servings.

If light cream is not available, substitute a mixture of equal parts milk and whipping cream.

Mousse au Chocolat

Just about the lightest mousse you've ever tasted!

4 egg yolks, room temperature
3/4 cup sugar
1/4 cup water
1 (6-oz.) pkg. semisweet chocolate pieces
   (1 cup)

1/2 cup butter
2 tablespoons almond-flavored liqueur or rum
4 egg whites, room temperature
1/4 teaspoon cream of tartar

In a small mixer bowl, beat egg yolks until thickened and lemon-colored. Heat sugar and water in a small saucepan until mixture begins to boil. Gradually pour hot mixture over egg yolks, beating constantly. Heat chocolate pieces and butter until chocolate melts. Stir in liqueur or rum; set aside. Place bowl with egg yolk mixture in a pan with almost boiling water. Beat egg yolk mixture 5 minutes or until doubled in volume. Remove from hot water; beat another 5 minutes. Pour into a large bowl. Fold chocolate mixture into egg yolk mixture. In a small bowl, beat egg whites with cream of tartar until stiff but not dry. Fold beaten egg whites into chocolate mixture. Spoon into a large serving bowl or dessert dishes. Refrigerate several hours. Makes 8 to 10 servings.

Orange Mousse

Shortcut mousse in a blender.

3 egg whites, room temperature
1/4 cup powdered sugar
4 oz. semisweet chocolate, coarsely chopped
3 tablespoons boiling water

3 egg yolks, room temperature
1 tablespoon orange liqueur
1 teaspoon grated orange peel
Whipped cream, if desired

In a medium mixing bowl, beat egg whites until soft peaks form. Gradually add powdered sugar. Beat until stiff; set aside. In blender container, combine chocolate and boiling water. Blend until smooth. Add egg yolks, liqueur and orange peel. Blend until smooth. Fold chocolate mixture into beaten egg whites. Spoon into sherbet glasses. Chill until firm. Garnish with whipped cream, if desired. Makes 4 or 5 servings.

Royal Pots de Crème

Easy to make but they're as good as dining at the King's palace.

4 oz. sweet cooking chocolate
2 tablespoons sugar
3/4 cup light cream

2 egg yolks, slightly beaten
1/2 teaspoon vanilla extract

Break chocolate into chunks. In a small saucepan over low heat, combine chocolate, sugar and cream. Stir constantly until smooth. Gradually pour over beaten egg yolks, beating constantly. Stir in vanilla. Pour into 5 or 6 pots de crème cups or custard cups. Chill. Makes 4 or 5 servings.

Pots de Crème au Chocolat

Vive le chocolat!

4 oz. semisweet chocolate	2 egg yolks
1 cup whipping cream	1 tablespoon vanilla extract
3 tablespoons sugar	Whipped cream, if desired
1 whole egg	

Preheat oven to 350°F (175°C). Break chocolate into small pieces. Combine cream and chocolate in a small saucepan. Heat over low heat, stirring until chocolate melts. Stir in sugar. In a medium bowl, slightly beat egg and egg yolks together. Add chocolate mixture gradually, stirring constantly. Stir in vanilla. Pour into 6 pots de crème cups or custard cups. Cover and set in a 13" x 9" baking pan. Pour boiling water into pan halfway up sides of cups. Bake on lower oven shelf 15 minutes or until almost firm. Remove cups from water; cool. Top with whipped cream, if desired. Makes 6 servings.

How To Make Pots de Crème au Chocolat

1/This type of Pots de Crème should be cooked like a custard. After adding chocolate and vanilla, pour mixture into Pots de Crème containers or custard cups that are placed in a 13" x 9" baking dish. If the containers have covers, be sure to use them. If not, cover each container with foil.

2/For best results, pour boiling water into the baking pan. This boiling water starts heating the mixture right away so the baking time is very short. To prevent overcooking, remove the cups from the water as soon as you take them out of the oven.

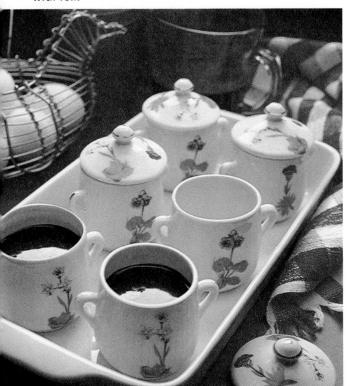

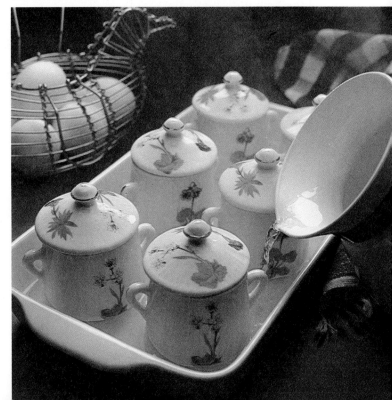

Easy Pots de Crème

A shortcut version with a hint of coffee.

3/4 cup milk
1 (6-oz.) pkg. semisweet chocolate pieces
  (1 cup)

2 eggs
2 tablespoons strong coffee
1 tablespoon orange-flavored liqueur

In a small saucepan, heat milk until small beads form around edges but do not boil. In blender container, combine chocolate pieces, eggs, coffee and liqueur. Blend until smooth. Add hot milk; blend again. Pour into 6 or 7 pots de crème cups or custard cups. Chill. Makes 6 or 7 servings.

Charlotte Russe

Light and airy, but rich with chocolate.

1 cup sugar
2 envelopes unflavored gelatin
3 oz. semisweet chocolate
2 cups milk
4 egg yolks, slightly beaten

3 tablespoons rum
15 ladyfingers, split lengthwise
4 egg whites
1 cup whipping cream (1/2 pint)
Additional whipped cream, if desired

In a small saucepan, combine sugar and gelatin. Add chocolate. Stir in milk and egg yolks. Stir constantly over low heat until smooth and slightly thickened. If flecks of chocolate remain, beat with a whisk or rotary beater. Pour into a large mixing bowl. Refrigerate, stirring occasionally, until gelatin begins to set. Sprinkle rum on ladyfingers. Stand about 18 ladyfinger halves upright around side of an 8-inch springform pan. In a large bowl, beat egg whites until stiff but not dry. Whip cream in a medium bowl. Fold egg whites into cooled chocolate mixture, then fold in whipped cream. Spoon half the mixture into pan lined with ladyfingers. Arrange remaining 12 ladyfinger halves over filling in mold. Top with remaining filling. Chill until firm. Unmold. Garnish with additional whipped cream, if desired. Makes 8 to 10 servings.

Molded Chocolate Cream

An impressive, habit-forming dessert.

7 whole ladyfingers, split lengthwise
4 oz. sweet cooking chocolate
3 tablespoons water
1 teaspoon grated orange peel

1 tablespoon orange-flavored liqueur
1 cup whipping cream
Whipped cream, if desired

Line bottom and sides of an 8" x 4" loaf pan with aluminum foil. Arrange a row of 6 ladyfinger halves along bottom of pan. Cut remaining 8 ladyfinger halves in half crosswise. Stand upright around sides of pan. In a small saucepan, combine chocolate, water and orange peel. Stir over low heat until melted. Cool. Stir in liqueur. Whip cream in a medium bowl. Fold chocolate mixture into whipped cream. Spoon into ladyfinger-lined pan. Chill several hours. To serve, lift from loaf pan onto serving plate. Peel off foil. Slice. Garnish with whipped cream, if desired. Makes 6 to 8 servings.

Soufflés & Cheesecakes

Soufflés have always had a mystical aura about them. Actually, there are two different kinds of soufflés. Both are delicately light because stiffly beaten egg whites are folded into the batter. Cold soufflés depend on gelatin to keep them airy and should be refrigerated several hours or overnight before serving. Hot soufflés depend on heat from the oven to make them rise, so timing is the key to successful hot soufflés. They must be served as soon as they are taken out of the oven.

Whether to beat egg whites in a copper bowl with a wire whisk, or in a mixer bowl with an electric beater is a controversial subject. A chemical reaction between the copper bowl and egg whites makes them more stable, so cream of tartar is not necessary. We have included cream of tartar in our recipes in case you use a non-copper bowl.

When making a dessert soufflé, first lightly oil the soufflé dish, then sprinkle it with sugar.

A collar gives an elegant look to a soufflé but is not necessary unless the soufflé mixture goes above the top of the dish. If you don't want to use a collar, use a larger soufflé dish.

To prepare a soufflé dish with a collar, lightly oil the soufflé dish and sprinkle with sugar. Tear off about 22 inches of aluminum foil for a 1-quart soufflé dish or 28 inches for the 6-cup size. Fold foil lengthwise in thirds to form a 22" or 28" x 4" strip. Lightly oil one side of the strip and sprinkle with sugar. Wrap around the soufflé dish with the oiled side inside, letting 1-1/2 to 2 inches of foil extend above top of the dish. Overlap ends and secure on the dish with tape or string. Fill with soufflé mixture and either bake or refrigerate, depending on the kind of soufflé. At serving time, carefully remove the collar.

Cheesecakes are not difficult, but you should allow enough time to make them and to let them cool properly.

If you haven't tried a chocolate cheesecake, you cannot understand why we are so enthusiastic about these irresistible desserts. We like them with chocolate in the filling, the crust, topping, or in all three. And we've added compatible flavors such as orange and mint to enhance the chocolate even more!

Fudge Soufflé

Light and airy with a deep fudge flavor.

3/4 cup sugar

1/2 cup flour

1-1/3 cups milk

6 oz. semisweet chocolate

2 tablespoons crème de cacao

6 egg yolks

6 egg whites

1/4 teaspoon cream of tartar

Powdered sugar

Prepare a 1-1/2-quart soufflé dish as described on page 89; set aside. Preheat oven to 325°F (165°C). In a medium saucepan, combine sugar and flour. Stir in milk. Stir constantly over low heat until thickened. Add chocolate; stir until smooth. Remove from heat. Stir in crème de cacao. In a medium mixing bowl, beat egg yolks until thickened and lemon-colored. Stir in chocolate mixture. In a large mixer bowl, beat egg whites until foamy. Add cream of tartar; beat until stiff but not dry. Fold about 1 cup beaten egg whites into chocolate mixture. Then fold chocolate mixture into remaining egg whites. Spoon into prepared soufflé dish. Bake about 1 hour and 5 minutes. Sprinkle with powdered sugar. Serve immediately. Makes 6 to 8 servings.

Mocha Soufflé

Guests will marvel at your culinary prowess.

1 cup milk

3 oz. semisweet chocolate, cut in small pieces

5 egg yolks

1/2 cup sugar

2 tablespoons flour

2 tablespoons cornstarch

1 tablespoon butter

1 tablespoon coffee-flavored liqueur

5 egg whites

1/4 teaspoon cream of tartar

Prepare a 1-1/2-quart soufflé dish as described on page 89; set aside. Preheat oven to 350°F (175°C). In a medium saucepan over low heat, combine milk and chocolate. Stir until chocolate melts. Remove from heat; set aside. In a medium mixing bowl, beat egg yolks until thickened and lemon-colored. Beat in sugar, flour and cornstarch until smooth. Add to melted chocolate in saucepan. Return saucepan to heat. Stir over low heat until mixture thickens. Remove from heat. Stir in butter and liqueur; set aside. In a large mixer bowl, beat egg whites until foamy. Add cream of tartar; continue beating until stiff peaks form. Fold in chocolate mixture. Spoon into prepared soufflé dish. Bake 45 minutes. Serve immediately. Makes 6 to 8 servings.

Coconut Soufflé

A delightfully flavored soufflé that holds up well.

4 oz. sweet cooking chocolate	1/3 cup whipping cream
6 egg yolks	1/2 cup flaked coconut
1/4 cup sugar	6 egg whites
1 (8-oz.) pkg. cream cheese, room temperature	1/4 teaspoon cream of tartar
1 (3-oz.) pkg. cream cheese, room temperature	

Melt chocolate; set aside. Prepare a 1-quart soufflé dish as described on page 89; set aside. Preheat oven to 350°F (175°C). In a medium mixing bowl, beat egg yolks until thickened and lemon-colored. Beat in sugar. Cut both packages of cream cheese into small cubes. Add to egg mixture; beat until smooth. Stir in cream, coconut and melted chocolate. In a large mixer bowl, beat egg whites until foamy. Add cream of tartar; continue beating until stiff but not dry. Stir about 1 cup of beaten egg whites into chocolate mixture; then gently fold chocolate mixture into remaining egg whites. Pour into prepared soufflé dish. Bake about 55 minutes. Serve immediately. Makes 6 to 8 servings.

Cocoa Soufflé

Remarkably beautiful!

2/3 cup sugar	1 teaspoon vanilla extract
1/3 cup unsweetened cocoa powder	4 egg yolks
3 tablespoons cornstarch	4 egg whites
3/4 cup milk	1/4 teaspoon cream of tartar
1/4 cup butter or margarine	Powdered sugar or sweetened whipped cream

Prepare a 1-quart soufflé dish as described on page 89, set aside. Preheat oven to 325°F (165°C). In a medium saucepan, combine sugar, cocoa and cornstarch. Gradually stir in milk. Stir constantly over low heat until mixture is thickened and smooth. Remove from heat. Stir in butter or margarine and vanilla; set aside to cool. In a medium mixing bowl, beat egg yolks until thickened and lemon-colored. Stir in cocoa mixture. In a large mixer bowl, beat egg whites until foamy. Add cream of tartar; continue beating until egg whites are stiff but not dry. Stir about 1 cup beaten egg whites into cocoa mixture, then gently fold cocoa mixture into remaining egg whites. Pour into prepared soufflé dish. Bake about 55 minutes. Serve immediately sprinkled with powdered sugar or topped with sweetened whipped cream. Makes 6 to 8 servings.

Be sure that egg whites are at room temperature when you beat them for soufflés.

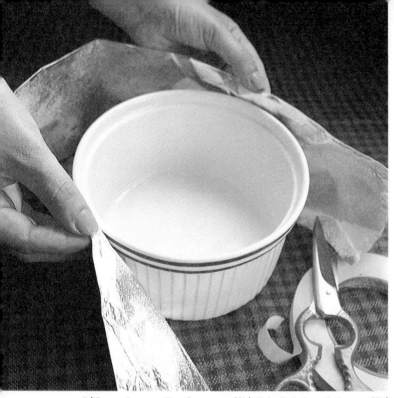

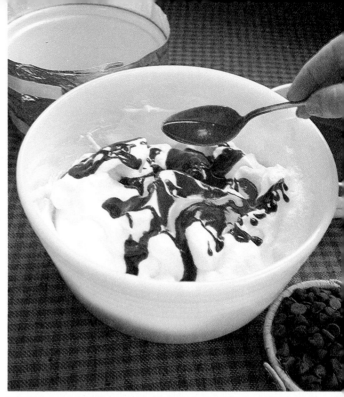

1/To make a collar for a soufflé dish, lightly oil the soufflé dish and sprinkle with sugar. For a 6-cup dish, fold a 28-inch-long piece of foil lengthwise into thirds. Lightly oil one side of the foil and sprinkle with sugar. Wrap the foil around the outside of the dish. Secure it with tape or string.

2/Set prepared dish aside. Cook and chill the chocolate mixture then fold the chilled mixture into stiffy beaten egg whites. Fold whipped cream into chocolate mixture. Spoon into prepared soufflé dish.

How To Make Crème de Cacao Soufflé

3/Allow plenty of time for the soufflé to set. Chill 6 hours or overnight so it will be thoroughly chilled and firm. Then carefully remove the foil collar by removing tape or string and slowly pulling foil away from chilled soufflé.

4/Just before serving, whip cream. Put in pastry bag with decorative tip. Form small mounds of cream around the edge and in the middle of the soufflé. Sprinkle with grated chocolate.

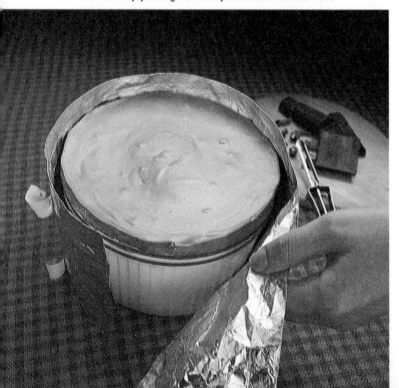

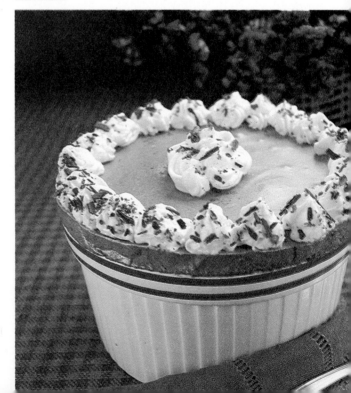

Crème de Cacao Soufflé

Cool elegance makes a lasting impression.

1/2 cup sugar
2 envelopes unflavored gelatin
1/4 teaspoon salt
1 cup water
6 egg yolks, slightly beaten
1 (6-oz.) pkg. semisweet chocolate pieces
   (1 cup)

1/3 cup crème de cacao
6 egg whites
1/2 cup sugar
1 cup whipping cream (1/2 pint)
Grated chocolate or chocolate curls
Whipped cream, if desired

Prepare a 6-cup soufflé dish with collar as shown on page 92; set aside. Mix 1/2 cup sugar, gelatin and salt in a medium saucepan. Stir in water. Add slightly beaten egg yolks and chocolate pieces. Stir constantly over medium heat until chocolate melts and mixture begins to simmer. Remove from heat; stir in crème de cacao. Chill until mixture mounds slightly when dropped from a spoon. In a large mixer bowl, beat egg whites until foamy. Gradually beat in 1/2 cup sugar; continue beating until stiff and glossy. Fold chilled chocolate mixture into beaten egg whites. In a medium bowl, beat 1 cup cream until stiff. Fold into chocolate mixture. Carefully spoon into prepared soufflé dish. Refrigerate 6 to 8 hours or until set. Just before serving, remove foil band. Garnish with grated chocolate or chocolate curls and whipped cream, if desired. Makes 10 to 12 servings.

Plantation Soufflé

What a cool refreshing way to end a meal!

1/4 cup cold water
1/3 cup crème de menthe
1 envelope unflavored gelatin
1/3 cup light brown sugar, lightly packed
1 (6-oz.) pkg. semisweet chocolate pieces
   (1 cup)

1/4 teaspoon salt
4 egg yolks
4 egg whites
1/3 cup light brown sugar, lightly packed
1 cup whipping cream (1/2 pint)

Combine water and crème de menthe in a medium saucepan. Sprinkle with gelatin. Add 1/3 cup brown sugar. Stir constantly over low heat until gelatin and sugar dissolve. Add chocolate pieces and salt. Stir until chocolate melts. Remove from heat. Stir in egg yolks 1 at a time. Cool. In a small bowl, beat egg whites until stiff but not dry. Gradually beat in 1/3 cup brown sugar; continue beating until very stiff peaks form. Fold into chocolate gelatin mixture. Whip cream; fold into chocolate-gelatin mixture. Turn into a 1-1/2 quart soufflé dish. Refrigerate several hours or overnight. Makes 6 servings.

Elegant Cheesecake

The ultimate in cheesecakes!

2 cups vanilla wafer crumbs (about 60 wafers)
2 tablespoons sugar
1/3 cup butter or margarine, melted
3 oz. semisweet chocolate
2 (8-oz.) pkgs. cream cheese,
    room temperature

1 cup sugar
4 egg yolks
1-1/2 cups dairy sour cream
1/4 cup flour
1-1/2 teaspoons vanilla extract
4 egg whites

In a medium bowl, mix crumbs, 2 tablespoons sugar and melted butter or margarine. Press on bottom and 2 inches up side of springform pan; refrigerate. Melt chocolate; set aside to cool. Preheat oven to 350°F (175°C). In a large mixer bowl, beat cream cheese and 1 cup sugar until light and creamy. Beat in egg yolks 1 at a time until blended. Stir sour cream into cooled chocolate. Add chocolate mixture, flour and vanilla to egg yolk mixture. Beat until smooth. In a small mixer bowl, beat egg whites until stiff but not dry. Fold into chocolate mixture. Spoon into prepared crust. Bake 55 to 60 minutes or until filling is firm. Turn off oven. Let cake cool in oven with door ajar 1 hour. Cool completely in pan on wire rack. Refrigerate several hours before cutting. Makes 10 to 12 servings.

Regal Cheesecake

Cottage cheese is the nutritious base for this tasty dessert.

2 cups graham cracker crumbs (28 crackers)
2 tablespoons sugar
1/3 cup butter or margarine, melted
2 cups cottage cheese
4 egg yolks
1 teaspoon vanilla extract
1/4 teaspoon almond extract

1-1/4 cups sugar
2/3 cup flour
1/2 teaspoon salt
2 oz. pre-melted unsweetened
    baking chocolate
1 cup dairy sour cream
4 egg whites

In a small bowl, mix cracker crumbs, 2 tablespoons sugar and melted butter or margarine. Set aside 1/4 cup mixture. Press remaining crumb mixture on bottom and about 1-1/2 to 2 inches up the side of a 9-inch springform pan; refrigerate. Preheat oven to 325°F (165°C). In a large mixer bowl, beat cottage cheese until curds are partially broken. Beat in egg yolks 1 at a time. Add vanilla and almond extracts, 1-1/4 cups sugar, flour and salt. Beat until blended. Beat in chocolate mixture and sour cream. In a small mixer bowl, beat egg whites until stiff but not dry. Fold into chocolate mixture. Pour into prepared crust. Sprinkle with 1/4 cup reserved crumb mixture. Bake 50 to 55 minutes. Turn off oven. Let cake cool in oven with door ajar 1 hour. Refrigerate several hours in pan. Remove side of pan. Cut cheesecake into wedges. Makes 10 to 12 servings.

Cocoa Cheesecake

A smooth chocolate cheesecake with sour cream topping.

1-1/2 cups zwieback crumbs
  (about 18 zwieback pieces)
2 tablespoons sugar
1/3 cup butter or margarine, melted
2 (8-oz.) pkgs. cream cheese,
  room temperature
1-1/4 cups sugar

1/3 cup unsweetened cocoa powder
1 teaspoon vanilla extract
2 eggs
1 cup dairy sour cream
2 tablespoons sugar
1/2 teaspoon vanilla extract

In a small bowl, combine crumbs, 2 tablespoons sugar and melted butter or margarine. Press on bottom and 1-1/2 to 2 inches up side of an 8-inch springform pan; refrigerate. Preheat oven to 375°F (190°C). In a medium mixing bowl, cream the cheese, 1-1/4 cups sugar and the cocoa. Add vanilla and eggs, beating until smooth. Pour into prepared crust. Bake 25 minutes. Remove from oven but do not turn off oven. In a small bowl, combine sour cream, 2 tablespoons sugar and vanilla. Spread over top of baked filling. Return to oven; bake 10 minutes. Cool several hours or overnight. Remove side of pan. Cut cheesecake into wedges. Makes 10 to 12 servings.

Grasshopper Cheesecake

You'll probably get more requests for this than for any other cheesecake.

1-1/2 cups chocolate cookie crumbs
  (about forty-two 1-1/2-inch chocolate snaps)
1 tablespoon sugar
2 tablespoons butter or margarine, melted
2 (8-oz.) pkgs. cream cheese,
  room temperature

1 cup sugar
3 eggs
1/4 cup green crème de menthe
2 tablespoons white crème de cacao
4 oz. sweet cooking chocolate
1/2 cup dairy sour cream

In a small bowl, combine crumbs, 1 tablespoon sugar and melted butter or margarine. Press on bottom and 1-1/2 inches up side of an 8-inch springform pan; refrigerate. Preheat oven to 350°F (175°C). In a large mixer bowl, cream the cheese and 1 cup sugar. Add eggs, beating until smooth. Stir in crème de menthe and crème de cacao. Pour into prepared crust. Bake 40 to 45 minutes. Cool in pan. Melt chocolate; cool about 5 minutes. Stir sour cream into melted chocolate. Spread over slightly cooled cheesecake. Refrigerate until set. Remove side of pan. Cut cheesecake into wedges and serve. Makes 8 to 10 servings.

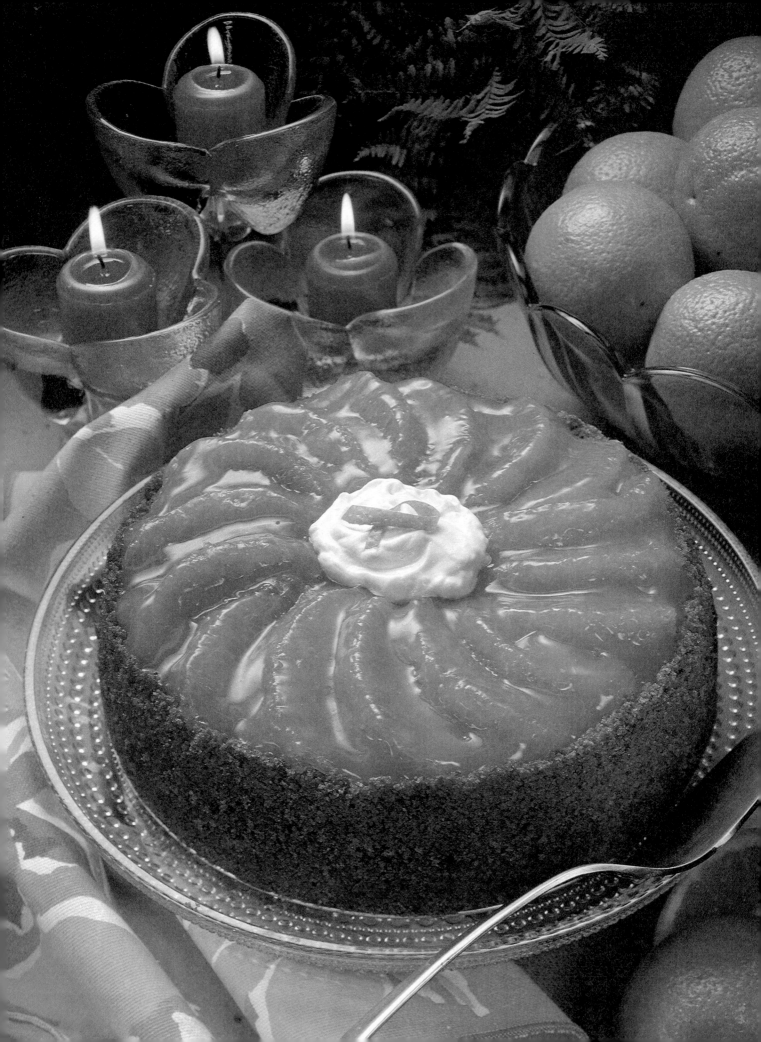

Orange-Glazed Cheesecake

Silky smooth texture and incredible flavor.

1-1/2 cups zwieback crumbs
  (about 18 zwieback pieces)
2 tablespoons sugar
1/4 teaspoon cinnamon
1/3 cup butter or margarine, melted
2 (8-oz.) pkgs. cream cheese,
  room temperature
1 cup sugar
1/4 cup unsweetened cocoa powder

1/4 teaspoon almond extract
2 eggs
1 cup dairy sour cream
1/3 cup sugar
2 tablespoons cornstarch
3/4 cup orange juice
1/4 cup orange-flavored liqueur
2 oranges, peeled and sectioned
Whipped cream, if desired

In a small bowl, combine zwieback crumbs, 2 tablespoons sugar, cinnamon and melted butter or margarine. Press on bottom and 1-1/2 inches up side of an 8-inch springform pan; refrigerate. Preheat oven to 350°F (175°C). In a large mixer bowl, cream the cheese, 1 cup sugar and the cocoa. Add almond extract and eggs, beating until smooth. Stir in sour cream. Pour into prepared crust. Bake 45 to 50 minutes. Cool in pan several hours. In a small saucepan, combine 1/3 cup sugar and cornstarch. Stir in orange juice. Bring to a boil over medium heat, stirring constantly. Simmer 1 minute longer. Remove glaze from heat. Add liqueur. Cool to lukewarm. Spoon half of glaze over cooled cheesecake. Arrange orange sections on top of glaze. Spoon remaining glaze over orange sections. Chill until firm. Remove side of pan. Garnish with whipped cream, if desired. Cut cheesecake into wedges. Makes 8 to 10 servings.

Cheesecakes are easier to cut if refrigerated overnight.

Tortes & Meringues

There may be arguments about the definition of a torte, but everyone agrees that tortes are not only a delicious dessert, but a dramatic one. To avoid confusion, we have grouped cake-type tortes with baked meringues.

If you enjoy the kind of torte that's made like a rich cake using ground nuts or crumbs for part or all of the flour, we have several of the best. If you are fond of the traditional European-type tortes, we hope you will try our version of Sacher Torte or Anne's Caramel Torte en Croûte.

Meringue tortes, sometimes called *Schaum Tortes,* are actually baked meringues. Unlike the meringue on a pie, these meringues contain more sugar, are beaten much stiffer and are baked longer at a lower temperature. The result is a hard meringue that is crumbly on the outside and slightly chewy in the middle. These meringues may be baked in a shell shape or flat in a cake pan. Or they may be combined with other ingredients to make a torte.

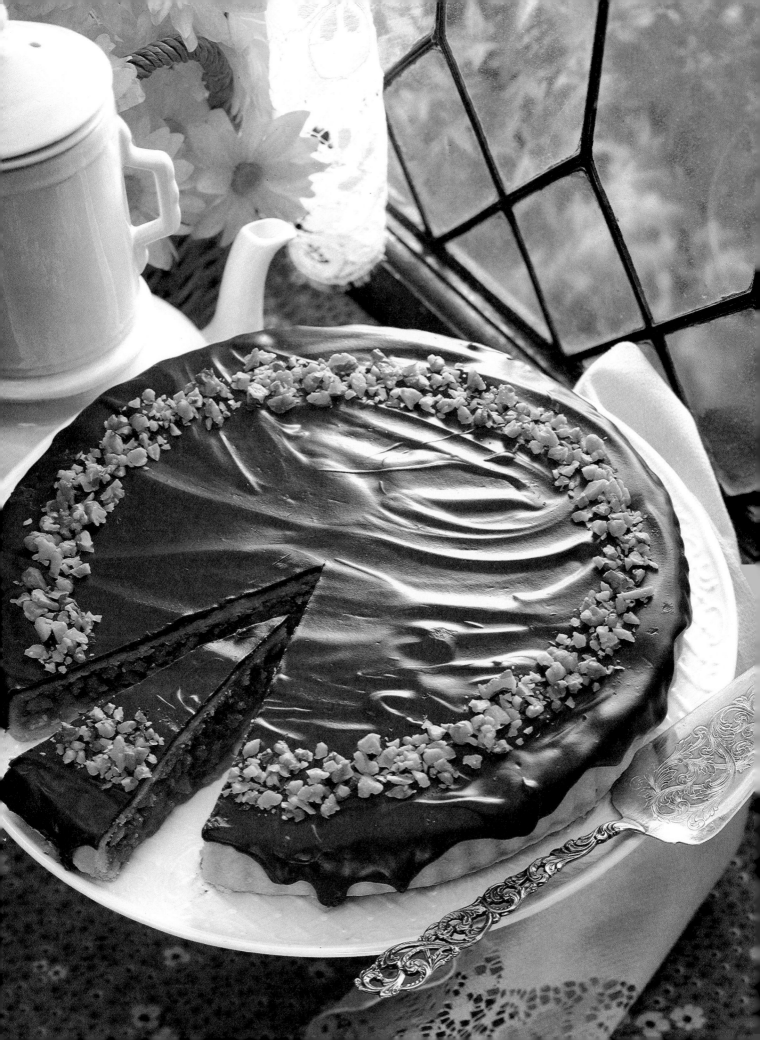

Anne's Caramel Torte en Croûte

Anne Otterson from the Perfect Pan shared this unusual torte recipe with us.

3-1/3 cups flour
1/4 cup sugar
1 cup cold butter, cut in small chunks
2 egg yolks, beaten slightly
6 tablespoons water
1-1/2 cups sugar
1/3 cup honey

1/2 cup water
3-1/2 cups chopped walnuts
1/4 cup butter
1 cup milk
Semisweet Glaze, see below
1/4 cup chopped walnuts

Semisweet Glaze:

1 (6-oz.) pkg. semisweet chocolate pieces
   (1 cup)

2 teaspoons cooking oil
1/4 cup unsalted butter

Butter a cookie sheet. Place outside ring of an 11-inch flan pan on the cookie sheet; set aside. In a large mixer bowl, combine flour with 1/4 cup sugar. Add 1 cup butter. Beat until mixture resembles soft fine breadcrumbs. Beat in egg yolks with 6 tablespoons water. By hand, quickly form into a ball and wrap in wax paper or aluminum foil. Refrigerate 30 minutes. Roll 2/3 of dough into a 12-1/2-inch circle. Refrigerate remaining dough. Fit rolled dough into flan ring on cookie sheet, leaving 1/2-inch overhang. Refrigerate 30 minutes. Combine 1-1/2 cups sugar, the honey and 1/2 cup water in a medium saucepan. Bring to a boil over medium heat. Cover; continue to boil 2 minutes. Remove cover. Boil uncovered over medium heat until mixture is a medium caramel color. Remove from heat. Stir in 3-1/2 cups chopped walnuts, 1/4 cup butter and milk. Return to heat; bring to a boil. Simmer over low heat 15 minutes, stirring occasionally. Preheat oven to 425°F (220°). To assemble, roll remaining 1/3 of dough into an 11-inch circle . Quickly pour filling into pastry-lined flan ring. Brush overhanging pastry edges with water. Place 11-inch circle of pastry over filling. Bring overhanging pastry over 11-inch circle; press lightly to seal. Cut slit in center. Bake 20 minutes. Let cool in ring on cookie sheet 4 hours. Invert cooled torte on a large serving plate. Remove flan ring. Prepare Semisweet Glaze. Pour glaze over top of torte, letting excess drip down sides. Sprinkle 1/4 cup chopped walnuts around top edge. Chill torte for easier cutting. Cut into wedges. Makes 12 to 14 servings.

Semisweet Glaze:
Melt chocolate pieces. Stir in oil and butter.

Egg whites for a baked meringue should be at room temperature and should be beaten until they are very stiff and glossy.

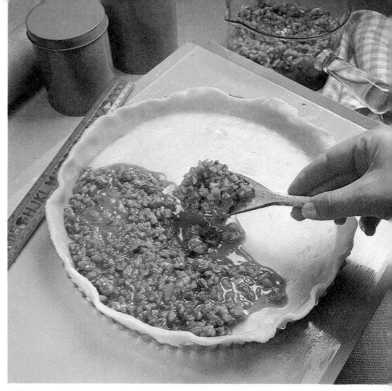

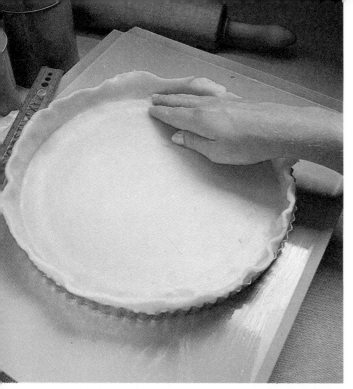

1/While pastry dough is refrigerating, place the ring of an 11-inch flan pan on a large buttered cookie sheet. Roll out 2/3 of the chilled dough into a 12-1/2-inch circle. Fit the circle into the bottom and over the sides of the flan ring. Allow about 1/2 inch overhang. Chill the pastry while you are making the filling.

2/Boil the sugar, honey and water until the mixture is caramel colored. Add walnuts, butter and milk. Simmer for another 15 minutes. Spoon filling into cooled pastry-lined pan.

How To Make Anne's Caramel Torte en Croûte

3/Roll remaining chilled pastry into an 11-inch circle. Place over filling in flan pan. Brush overhanging pastry with water, then fold it over the 11-inch pastry circle. Gently press edges to seal. You don't have to worry about neat edges because this will be the bottom of torte. Cut a slit in the center of the pastry and bake.

4/After torte is baked, let it cool on the cookie sheet about 4 hours. Then invert it onto a large serving plate and remove the flan ring. Spread the torte with glaze and sprinkle with nuts. This torte is quite rich so you can serve it in small slices.

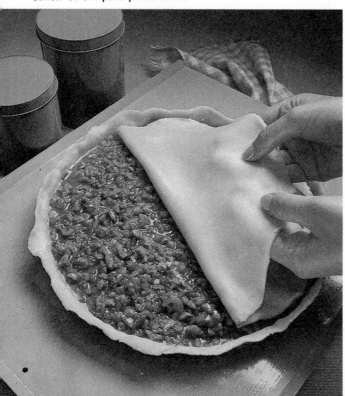

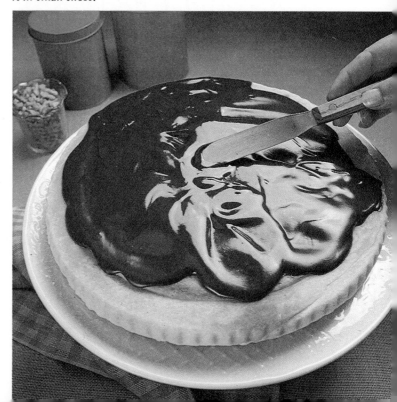

Sacher Torte

One of the most famous European tortes.

4 oz. semisweet chocolate	3/4 cup flour
3/4 cup butter or margarine	5 egg whites
3/4 cup sugar	1/2 cup apricot jam
5 egg yolks	Honey Glaze, see below

Honey Glaze:

2 oz. unsweetened chocolate	1 tablespoon honey
2 oz. semisweet chocolate	1/4 cup butter

Melt chocolate; set aside. Grease and flour a 9-inch springform pan; set aside. Preheat oven to 325°F (165°C). In a large mixer bowl, cream butter or margarine and sugar until creamy. Add egg yolks 1 at a time, beating until light and fluffy. Mix in melted chocolate. Gradually beat in flour. In a medium mixing bowl, beat egg whites until stiff but not dry. Fold into chocolate mixture. Spoon into prepared pan. Bake 50 to 60 minutes. Let stand in pan on cooling rack 10 minutes. Remove outside ring of pan. Cool cake on rack. Strain apricot jam. When cake is cool, split horizontally. Spread strained jam on bottom layer. Replace top layer. Prepare Honey Glaze. Spoon over top of cooled cake, letting excess drip down sides. Makes 8 to 10 servings.

Honey Glaze:
In a small saucepan over very low heat, melt unsweetened chocolate and semisweet chocolate with honey and butter. Stir until smooth. Remove from heat. Stir over ice water until slightly thickened and syrupy.

Almond-Cherry Squares

Watch this three-flavored torte disappear!

1/2 cup blanched almonds	1/8 teaspoon cream of tartar
4 oz. semisweet chocolate	2 tablespoons sugar
1/4 cup butter or margarine	1 cup sweet, dark pitted canned cherries,
1/3 cup sugar	well-drained
4 egg yolks	Whipped cream
4 egg whites	

Grind almonds in a food chopper or blender. set aside. Melt chocolate; set aside. Grease and flour an 8-inch square baking pan; set aside. Preheat oven to 350°F (175°C). In a medium mixing bowl, cream butter or margarine and 1/3 cup sugar until fluffy. Beat in egg yolks. Stir in melted chocolate and ground almonds. In a small mixer bowl, beat egg whites and cream of tartar until foamy. Gradually add 2 tablespoons sugar; beat until stiff but not dry. Fold into chocolate mixture. Pour into prepared pan. Spoon well-drained cherries over top. Bake 20 to 25 minutes. Cool before cutting into 2-inch squares. Top squares with whipped cream. Makes 16 servings.

Walnut Torte

A traditional French torte adapted to contemporary taste.

5 oz. semisweet chocolate
1-1/2 cups walnuts
2 tablespoons sugar
2 tablespoons flour
3/4 cup butter

1/2 cup sugar
5 egg yolks
5 egg whites
Chocolate Whipped Cream, see below
Walnut halves, if desired

Chocolate Whipped Cream:
4 oz. sweet cooking chocolate
1 cup whipping cream (1/2 pint)

1/2 teaspoon vanilla extract

Melt chocolate; set aside. Grease and flour a 9-inch springform pan; set aside. Preheat oven to 350°F (175°C). Place walnuts, 2 tablespoons sugar and flour in blender container; blend until walnuts are finely ground. In a large mixer bowl, cream butter. Add 1/2 cup sugar; beat until light. Add egg yolks 1 at a time, beating well after each addition. Stir in melted chocolate, then nut mixture. In a large mixer bowl, beat egg whites until stiff. Fold into chocolate batter. Spoon into prepared pan. Bake about 40 minutes. Cool in pan on wire rack 10 minutes. Remove side of pan. Cool completely on rack. Prepare Chocolate Whipped Cream. Spread on top of cooled cake. Garnish with walnut halves, if desired. Makes 8 to 10 servings.

Chocolate Whipped Cream:
Melt chocolate; cool to lukewarm. Beat cream until stiff. Stir in vanilla. Fold cooled chocolate into whipped cream.

Mint Dreams

Truly a heavenly dessert.

3 egg whites
1/8 teaspoon salt
3/4 cup sugar
1/2 teaspoon vanilla extract
3/4 cup fine chocolate wafer crumbs

1/2 cup chopped walnuts
1 cup whipping cream
2 tablespoons sugar
1/2 cup crushed peppermint candy
1 oz. semisweet chocolate, grated

Grease a 9-inch square baking pan; set aside. Preheat oven to 325°F (165°C). In a medium mixing bowl, beat egg whites and salt until soft peaks form. Gradually add 3/4 cup sugar, beating until glossy and stiff peaks form. Beat in vanilla. Fold in crumbs and walnuts. Spread in prepared pan. Bake 35 minutes. Cool. Several hours before serving, whip cream. Fold in 2 tablespoons sugar and peppermint candy. Spread over cooled chocolate mixture. Garnish with grated chocolate. Cut into squares. Makes 9 servings.

Dobos Torte

You'll need 6 layers, so reuse your cake pans while the first layers are cooling.

1 cup butter, room temperature

1 cup sugar

4 whole eggs

1-1/2 cups flour

1 teaspoon vanilla extract

4 oz. unsweetened chocolate

1 cup sugar

1/4 teaspoon cream of tartar

1/2 cup water

6 egg yolks

1 cup butter, room temperature

2/3 cup sugar

1/3 cup water

Grease and flour 9-inch cake pans; set aside. Preheat oven to 350°F (175°C). In a large mixer bowl, cream 1 cup butter and 1 cup sugar until light and fluffy. Beat in whole eggs, then stir in flour and vanilla until batter is smooth. Spoon about 2/3 cup batter about 1/8 inch thick into each prepared pan. Bake 7 to 9 minutes or until lightly browned around edges. Remove from pan. Cool on wire rack. Repeat until all batter is used and you have 6 cool layers. Melt chocolate; set aside. In a medium saucepan, combine 1 cup sugar, cream of tartar and 1/2 cup water. Stir over low heat until sugar dissolves. Boil on moderate heat without stirring until syrup reaches 283°F (115°C) on a candy thermometer or soft-ball stage. While syrup is cooking, beat egg yolks in a medium bowl until thick and lemon-colored. Gradually pour hot syrup over beaten eggs, beating until mixture is lukewarm and creamy. Beat in 1 cup butter, then melted chocolate. Spread a thin layer of filling between cake layers but not on top layer. In a small heavy saucepan, combine 2/3 cup sugar and 1/3 cup water. Cook over moderate heat without stirring until sugar dissolves and begins to darken, 10 to 12 minutes. Occasionally swirling the pan, continue to boil until glaze becomes golden brown. Immediately pour glaze over top layer. With a buttered knife, quickly mark glaze into 12 to 16 equal wedges, cutting almost but not quite through the glaze. Refrigerate several hours or overnight. Makes 10 to 12 servings.

To fold beaten egg whites into a very heavy or thick batter, first fold a small amount of the egg whites into the batter to lighten it, then fold in the remaining egg whites.

Orange-Chocolate Torte

A meringue-like torte laced with graham cracker crumbs and nuts.

About 14 graham crackers	1 cup sugar
1 cup walnuts	1 teaspoon grated orange peel
3 egg whites	1/2 cup semisweet chocolate pieces
1/4 teaspoon cream of tartar	Orange-Chocolate Glaze, see below

Orange-Chocolate Glaze:

1/2 cup semisweet chocolate pieces	1/2 cup dairy sour cream
1/2 cup milk chocolate pieces	2 tablespoons orange-flavored liqueur

Butter a 9-inch springform pan; set aside. Preheat oven to 350°F (175°C). In a blender, pulverize enough graham crackers to make 1 cup of fine crumbs. Remove from blender; set aside. Pulverize nuts into fine crumbs; set aside. In a medium mixing bowl, beat egg whites and cream of tartar until foamy. Gradually add sugar, beating until stiff and glossy. Fold in graham cracker crumbs, walnut crumbs and orange peel, then chocolate pieces. Bake 25 to 30 minutes. Cool in pan. Remove from pan. Prepare Orange-Chocolate Glaze. Spread on cooled torte, letting excess drip down sides. Cut in wedges. Makes 6 servings.

Orange-Chocolate Glaze:

In top of a double boiler over hot but not boiling water, melt semisweet and milk chocolate pieces, stirring until smooth. Stir in sour cream and liqueur.

Meringue Torte

Like eating a cloud!

5 egg whites	2 tablespoons powdered sugar
1 teaspoon vanilla extract	1 tablespoon unsweetened cocoa powder
1-1/4 cups granulated sugar	Grated chocolate, if desired
1 cup whipping cream (1/2 pint)	

Line 2 large cookie sheets with brown paper. Draw two 9-inch circles on one paper and one 9-inch circle on the other; set aside. Preheat oven to 250°F (120°C). In a large bowl, beat egg whites until soft peaks form. Add vanilla. Gradually add granulated sugar, beating until very thick and glossy. Spoon beaten egg whites onto each circle; spread inside circle with a spatula. Bake 40 to 45 minutes or until very lightly colored and crisp. Cool about 10 minutes. Very carefully lift meringues off paper; cool. In a medium mixing bowl, beat cream until it begins to thicken. Gradually beat in powdered sugar. Fold in cocoa. Stack baked meringues with cream filling between each meringue and on top. Refrigerate several hours. Garnish with grated chocolate, if desired. Makes 10 to 12 servings.

Minted Cocoa Meringues

Mint cream spread between chocolate meringues and topped with your favorite chocolate sauce.

3 egg whites
1/4 teaspoon cream of tartar
3/4 cup sugar
3 tablespoons unsweetened cocoa powder
1 cup whipping cream

2 tablespoons sugar
2 tablespoons crème de menthe
Several drops green food coloring
Royal Chocolate Sauce, page 36

Line 2 cookie sheets with brown paper; set aside. Preheat oven to 275°F (135°C). In a medium mixing bowl, beat egg whites and cream of tartar until foamy. Gradually beat in 3/4 cup sugar. Continue beating until very stiff and glossy. Sprinkle cocoa over mixture. Continue beating until blended. Attach a large star tip to a pastry tube. Fill tube with cocoa mixture. Make twenty 2- to 2-1/2-inch meringues on brown paper. Bake 30 minutes. Turn off oven; leave meringues in oven for an hour with door closed. Remove from oven and cool. In a medium mixing bowl, beat cream until it begins to thicken. Gradually add 2 tablespoons sugar, crème de menthe and green food coloring. Beat until stiff. Put flat sides of 2 meringues together with about 2 heaping tablespoons of cream in between. Place filled meringues on their sides. Refrigerate several hours. Prepare Royal Chocolate Sauce. At serving time, spoon chocolate sauce over each filled meringue. Makes 10 servings.

Meringue Mushrooms

For best results, make these on a dry day. Use to decorate desserts or fill a pretty centerpiece basket.

3 egg whites
1/4 teaspoon cream of tartar
2/3 cup sugar

1/2 cup semisweet or milk chocolate pieces
Unsweetened cocoa powder

Line a baking sheet with parchment paper; set aside. Preheat oven to 225°F (105°C). In a small mixer bowl, beat egg whites until foamy. Add cream of tartar. Beat until soft peaks form. Add sugar gradually, beating until very stiff peaks form. Place meringue in a pastry bag with a large plain tip, 1/2 inch in diameter. To make caps: On prepared baking sheet, pipe out small mounds of meringue 1- to 1-1/2 inches in diameter. Smooth tops with a spatula. To make stems: Holding pastry bag vertically and placing stems about 1 inch from caps, pipe out stems 1-1/2 inches long. Bake 1 to 1-1/4 hours or until thoroughly dry. Cool. Remove from pan. Melt chocolate pieces. To assemble mushrooms: With a small knife, cut a hole in bottom of cap to fit stem into. Spread a layer of chocolate over bottom of cap. Place one end of stem on chocolate in hole. Let stand upside down or on side on cooling rack or in empty egg carton until chocolate hardens. Repeat with remaining caps and stems. If desired, refrigerate a few minutes but do not freeze. Sift cocoa over mushrooms to resemble real mushrooms. Cover and store at room temperature. Makes about 20 mushrooms.

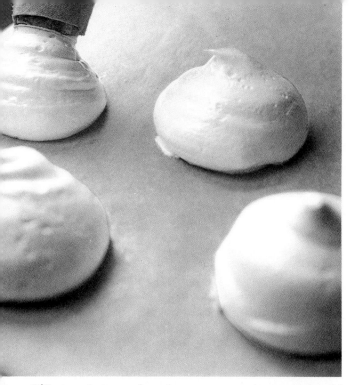

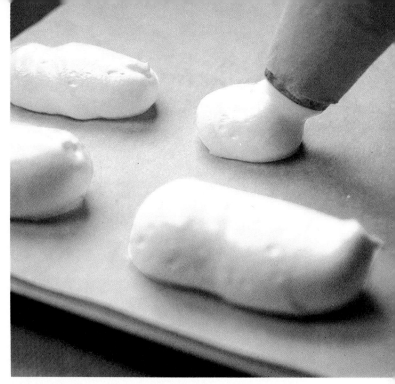

1/Caps and stems of mushrooms are made separately and then put together after they are baked. To make caps, place meringue mixture in a pastry bag with a large plain tip. Push out 1- to 1-1/2-inch mounds of meringue onto the parchment-lined cookie sheet. Cut off any peaks or smooth tops with a small spatula.

2/To make stems, place meringue mixture in the pastry bag with a large plain tip. On parchment-lined cookie sheet, push out stems about 1-1/2 inches long and about 3/4 inch wide. Smooth any peaks with a small spatula. Make an equal number of stems and caps.

How To Make Meringue Mushrooms

3/Bake caps and stems until thoroughly dry. When completely cooled, put together. Hold one cap upside down and cut a small hole out of the center. This hole is for the stem to fit into. Then spread a layer of melted chocolate into the hole and over half the bottom of the cap. Immediately place one end of the stem into the chocolate-coated hole. Let mushrooms stand on rack until chocolate hardens.

4/If the chocolate holding mushrooms together does not harden at room temperature, refrigerate the mushrooms for a few minutes. After the chocolate is firm, place a small amount of unsweetened cocoa powder in a strainer or sifter. Lightly sift cocoa over the mushrooms so they have a realistic look. Use to decorate cakes or as a centerpiece.

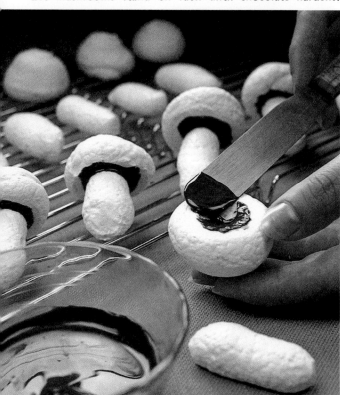

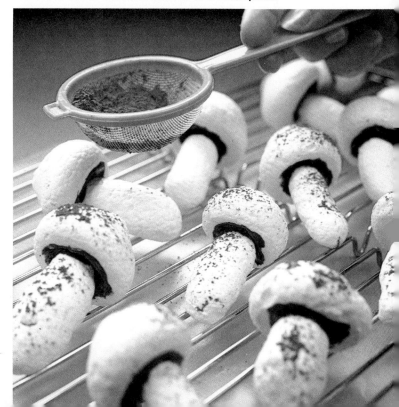

Pies & Pie Crusts

When you want a chocolate pie, do you make a rich chocolate meringue pie, a light and airy chiffon or a fudge cream pie? We've included all of these — and many more.

One of our favorites is No-Crust Brownie Pie. Similar to a brownie, but made in a pie pan without a crust, it's a quick and easy dessert you can make ahead of time and serve with ice cream.

You can mix or match pie crusts and fillings. That is, fill a chocolate crust with chocolate filling, or make a regular pie crust for the base of a Grasshopper Pie or Black Bottom Pie.

When making pie fillings with chocolate, milk and eggs, use heat in moderation. Chocolate scorches easily so the mixture needs to be watched carefully and stirred frequently. In case the filling you cooked on top of the stove still has flecks of chocolate in it, beat it slightly with a wire whisk or hand mixer before pouring it into the pie shell.

Whipped cream is the crowning glory for many chocolate pies. Just before serving, whip the cream and spoon it on top of the pie. For a more elegant look, put the whipped cream in a pastry tube and pipe a wide ruffle around the pie's edge or make rosettes on each slice. A sprinkle of grated chocolate makes a decorative finishing touch.

Toffee-Coffee Pie

One of our very favorites!

1 stick pie crust mix
1/4 cup light brown sugar, firmly packed
3/4 cup chopped walnuts
1 oz. unsweetened chocolate, grated
1 teaspoon vanilla extract
1 tablespoon water

1 oz. unsweetened chocolate
1/2 cup butter, room temperature
3/4 cup granulated sugar
2 teaspoons instant coffee powder
2 eggs
Coffee Cream Topping, see below

Coffee Cream Topping:
1 cup whipping cream (1/2 pint)
2 teaspoons instant coffee powder

1 tablespoon powdered sugar

Butter an 8-inch pie pan. Preheat oven to 375°F (190°C). In a medium bowl, crumble pie crust stick with a pastry blender or fork until very fine. Blend in brown sugar, walnuts and 1 ounce grated chocolate. Sprinkle 1 tablespoon of mixture in a shallow baking pan; set aside. Add vanilla and water to remaining mixture; mix well. Press firmly into bottom and on side of prepared pan. Moisten fingers with cold water for easier handling. Bake 15 minutes. Also bake reserved 1 tablespoon pastry crumbs in baking pan 5 minutes. Cool crust and crumbs. Melt 1 ounce chocolate; set aside to cool. In a medium mixing bowl, cream butter. Add granulated sugar gradually, beating until light and fluffy. Stir in cooled chocolate and instant coffee powder. Add eggs 1 at a time, beating 5 minutes after each addition. Pour into cooled crust. Prepare Coffee Cream Topping. Spread on top of filling. Sprinkle with reserved baked crumbs. Refrigerate 2 hours before serving. Makes one 8-inch pie.

Coffee Cream Topping:
In a small mixer bowl, beat cream until it begins to thicken. Gradually add instant coffee powder and powdered sugar, beating until stiff.

When putting meringue on a pie filling, push the meringue against the pie crust so it will seal while baking.

Chocolate Cream Pie

A no-fuss pie you can depend on.

1 cup sugar

1/4 cup cornstarch

1/4 teaspoon salt

1-1/2 cups cold water

3 eggs, slightly beaten

3 oz. semisweet chocolate, broken in chunks

2 tablespoons butter or margarine

1 teaspoon vanilla extract

1 (9-inch) pie shell, baked

1/2 cup whipping cream

In a medium saucepan, mix sugar, cornstarch and salt. Pour in water. Stir until blended. Add eggs and chocolate. Stir constantly over low heat until thickened and smooth. Remove from heat; stir in butter or margarine and vanilla. Pour into baked pie shell. Refrigerate several hours or until firm. Whip cream; spread over pie. Makes one 9-inch pie.

Fudge Meringue Pie

Enjoy the delicious fudge-like filling.

1 cup sugar

1/3 cup flour

1/4 teaspoon salt

2 cups milk

2 oz. unsweetened chocolate,
   broken in small chunks

3 egg yolks, slightly beaten

2 tablespoons butter or margarine

1 teaspoon vanilla extract

1 (9-inch) pie shell, baked and cooled

3 egg whites

1/2 teaspoon vanilla extract

1/4 teaspoon cream of tartar

6 tablespoons sugar

In a medium saucepan, combine 1 cup sugar, the flour and salt. Gradually stir in milk. Add chocolate. Stir constantly over medium heat until bubbly. Simmer 2 minutes longer. Remove from heat. Stir a small amount of hot mixture into beaten egg yolks; immediately add egg yolk mixture to remaining hot mixture in saucepan. Stir constantly over medium heat 2 minutes. Remove from heat. Add butter or margarine and 1 teaspoon vanilla. Pour into cooled baked pie shell. Preheat oven to 350°F (175°C). In a small bowl, beat egg whites, 1/2 teaspoon vanilla and cream of tartar until foamy. Gradually beat in 6 tablespoons sugar, beating until stiff and glossy. Spoon meringue on chocolate filling, carefully sealing to edge of crust. Bake 12 to 15 minutes or until golden. Cool. Makes 6 to 8 servings.

Refrigerate a chocolate chiffon pie several hours so it will be firm enough to cut.

Sour Cream Meringue Pie

A welcome finale to a hearty supper!

1 cup light brown sugar, lightly packed
2 tablespoons flour
1/4 teaspoon cinnamon
1 cup dairy sour cream
3 egg yolks, slightly beaten
2 tablespoons butter or margarine, melted

1 teaspoon vanilla extract
1 (6-oz.) semisweet chocolate pieces (1 cup)
1 (9-inch) unbaked pie shell
3 egg whites
1/4 teaspoon cream of tartar
1/3 cup granulated sugar

Preheat oven to 375°F (190°C). In a large bowl, combine brown sugar, flour, cinnamon, sour cream, egg yolks, melted butter or margarine and vanilla. Beat until smooth. Stir in chocolate pieces; mix well. Pour into unbaked pie shell. Bake 45 to 50 minutes or until tip of knife inserted in center comes out clean. In a medium bowl, beat egg whites and cream of tartar until foamy. Gradually add granulated sugar. Continue beating until stiff peaks form. Spread meringue over warm pie filling, carefully sealing to edge of crust. Bake 7 to 10 minutes or until golden. Cool on wire rack 1 hour. Serve slightly warm. Makes one 9-inch pie.

Chocolate Banana Cream Pie

It's hard to beat this chocolate-banana blend!

1/2 cup sugar
1/2 teaspoon salt
1/3 cup cornstarch
2-1/2 cups milk
1 (6-oz.) pkg. semisweet chocolate pieces
   (1 cup)

1 teaspoon vanilla extract
3 egg yolks, slightly beaten
1 (9-inch) pie shell, baked
2 medium bananas
1/2 cup whipping cream

In a medium saucepan, stir together sugar, salt and cornstarch. Gradually stir in milk. Add chocolate pieces and vanilla. Bring to a boil over medium heat, stirring constantly. Continue stirring and boiling 1 minute longer. Remove from heat. Stir a little hot mixture into egg yolks; mix well. Add egg yolk mixture to remaining hot mixture in saucepan. Stir over low heat 5 minutes or until thickened. Pour half of mixture into baked pie shell. Peel bananas and slice crosswise. Layer slices over filling in pie shell; cover with remaining filling, spreading evenly. Place wax paper directly on surface of filling. Refrigerate until set, 3 to 4 hours. Before serving, whip cream and use to garnish edge of pie. Makes one 9-inch pie.

Chocolate Chiffon Pie

Rich with chocolate, yet so light.

1 envelope unflavored gelatin
1/2 cup sugar
1/2 teaspoon salt
1-1/3 cups milk
3 oz. semisweet chocolate, broken in chunks
3 egg yolks

1 teaspoon vanilla extract
3 egg whites
1/4 teaspoon cream of tartar
1/2 cup sugar
1 (9-inch) pie shell, baked
Whipped cream, if desired

In a medium saucepan, combine gelatin, 1/2 cup sugar and salt. Gradually stir in milk. Add chocolate. Place over low heat until chocolate melts. Remove from heat. In a small bowl, beat egg yolks slightly. Stir a small amount of chocolate mixture into egg yolks. Then add egg yolk mixture to remaining chocolate mixture in saucepan. Stir constantly until thickened. Stir in vanilla. Cool until mixture mounds when dropped from a spoon. In a medium bowl, beat egg whites and cream of tartar until foamy. Gradually add 1/2 cup sugar. Beat until stiff but not dry. Fold into cooled chocolate mixture. Pour into baked pie shell. Refrigerate several hours. Top with whipped cream, if desired. Makes one 9-inch pie.

Peanut Crunch Pie

Every bite is an exciting treat!

1-1/2 cups ground peanuts
1/4 cup sugar
2 tablespoons butter or margarine,
 room temperature
1-1/2 cups miniature marshmallows or
 16 large marshmallows

1/2 cup milk
1 (8-oz.) milk chocolate candy bar
1 cup whipping cream (1/2 pint)

Preheat oven to 400°F (205°C). In a small mixer bowl, thoroughly combine peanuts, sugar and butter or margarine. Press mixture firmly and evenly against bottom and side of a 9-inch pie pan. Bake 6 to 8 minutes; cool. In a medium saucepan, combine marshmallows, milk and chocolate bar. Stir constantly over low heat until chocolate and marshmallows are melted and mixture is smooth. Refrigerate, stirring occasionally, until mixture mounds slightly when dropped from a spoon. In a small mixer bowl, beat whipping cream until stiff. Fold into chocolate mixture. Pour into cooled prepared pie shell. Refrigerate until set, about 8 hours. Makes one 9-inch pie.

Almond-Marshmallow Pie

Imagine all your favorite flavors in one pie!

1-1/2 cups finely crushed vanilla wafer
   crumbs (about 42 wafers)
1 teaspoon cinnamon
1/4 cup butter or margarine, melted
20 large marshmallows

1 (8-oz.) milk chocolate candy bar
2/3 cup milk
1/3 cup sliced almonds
1/2 cup whipping cream

Preheat oven to 350°F (175°C). In a small mixing bowl, combine crumbs, cinnamon and melted butter or margarine. Pat into a 9-inch pie pan. Bake 10 minutes. Cool. In a medium saucepan, combine marshmallows, chocolate bar and milk. Place over low heat until marshmallows and chocolate bar are melted. Cool. Preheat oven to 300°F (150°C). Toast almonds on baking sheet in oven about 20 minutes, stirring once or twice. Whip cream; fold into chocolate mixture. Pour into prepared pie shell. Sprinkle with toasted almonds. Chill and serve. Makes one 9-inch pie.

Chocolate Buttercream Pie

Reminiscent of those famous French buttercreams.

4 oz. unsweetened chocolate
3/4 cup butter
1 cup sugar
2 teaspoons vanilla extract

4 eggs
1 (9-inch) pie shell, baked
Whipped cream, if desired

Melt chocolate; set aside to cool. In a small mixer bowl, cream butter. Add sugar, melted chocolate and vanilla. Beat until light and fluffy. Add eggs. Beat about 3 minutes, until mixture is smooth and thick. Pour into baked pie shell; chill. Garnish with whipped cream, if desired. Makes one 9-inch pie.

Grasshopper Pie

The most popular choice for a dinner party.

1-1/2 cups chocolate cookie crumbs
   (24 thin chocolate wafers)
1 tablespoon sugar
2 tablespoons butter or margarine, melted
32 large marshmallows
1/2 cup milk

1/4 cup green crème de menthe
3 tablespoons white crème de cacao
1 cup whipping cream (1/2 pint)
Whipped cream, if desired
Grated chocolate, if desired

Combine crumbs, sugar and melted butter or margarine. Press on bottom and side of a 9-inch pie pan. Refrigerate while making filling. In a medium saucepan, combine marshmallows and milk. Stir constantly over low heat until marshmallows melt. Refrigerate until thickened. Stir in crème de menthe and crème de cacao. In a medium bowl, beat cream until stiff. Fold in cool marshmallow mixture. Pour into prepared crust. Refrigerate until firm. If desired, garnish with whipped cream and grated chocolate. Makes one 9-inch pie.

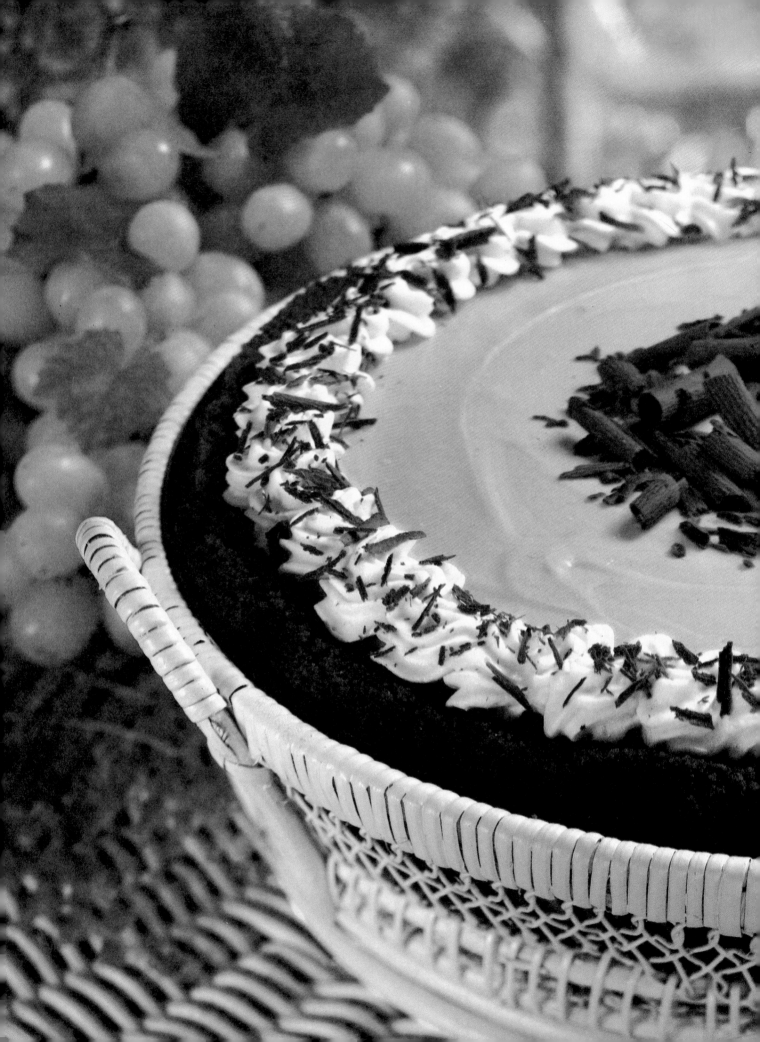

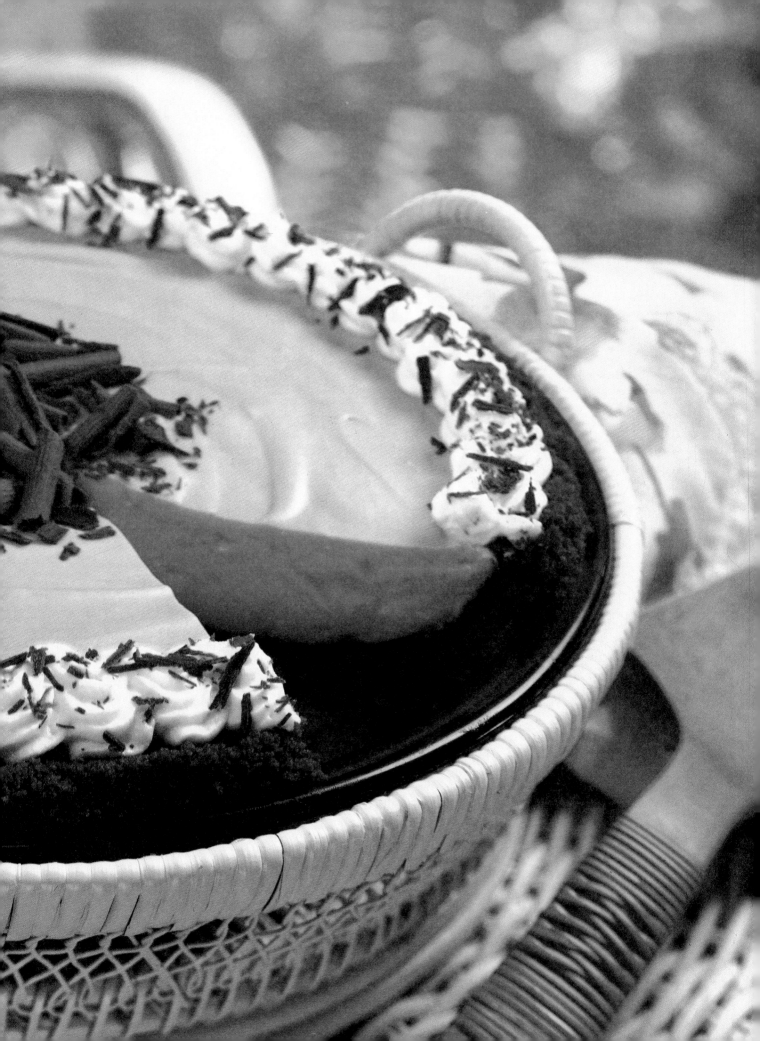

Pecan Pie

Chocolate adds distinctive flavor to a traditional pie.

1 (9-inch) unbaked pie shell
1-1/4 cups light corn syrup
1/2 cup sugar
4-oz. sweet cooking chocolate

1/2 cup evaporated milk, not diluted
3 eggs, slightly beaten
1 cup pecan halves

Crimp edge of pie shell so it stands high and will hold the entire amount of filling; set aside. Preheat oven to 350°F (175°C). In a medium saucepan, combine corn syrup, sugar, chocolate and evaporated milk. Stir constantly over low heat until chocolate just melts. Very gradually stir hot mixture into beaten eggs, then stir in pecans. Pour into unbaked pie shell. Bake 50 to 60 minutes or until fairly firm. Center will be slightly soft but will become firmer as pie cools. Makes one 9-inch pie.

No-Crust Brownie Pie

Absolute bliss served a la mode, but delicious all by itself.

2 eggs, well-beaten
1 cup sugar
1/2 cup butter, melted
1/2 cup flour
5 tablespoons unsweetened cocoa powder

1/4 teaspoon salt
1 teaspoon vanilla extract
1 cup chopped walnuts
Ice cream or whipped cream, if desired

Lightly grease an 8-inch pie pan; set aside. Preheat oven to 350°F (175°C). In a medium bowl, mix eggs with sugar and melted butter. Stir together flour, cocoa and salt. Add to egg mixture. Stir in vanilla and nuts. Pour into prepared pie pan without a pie shell. Bake 20 to 25 minutes. Cool before cutting into wedges. Serve plain, with ice cream or with whipped cream. Makes one 8-inch pie.

Black Bottom Pie

Light and airy on top with rich chocolate underneath.

1 tablespoon unflavored gelatin
1/4 cup cold water
1 tablespoon cornstarch
1/2 cup sugar
1-1/2 cups milk
3 egg yolks, slightly beaten
1 (1-oz.) pkg. pre-melted unsweetened
   baking chocolate

1 teaspoon vanilla extract
1 (9-inch) pie shell, baked
1 tablespoon rum
3 egg whites
1/3 cup sugar
Whipped cream, if desired
Grated chocolate, if desired

Sprinkle gelatin over water; stir and set aside. In a medium saucepan, combine cornstarch and 1/2 cup sugar. Stir in milk. Cook over low heat until mixture is slightly thickened and translucent. Remove from heat. Stir about half of milk mixture into beaten egg yolks. Add egg yolk mixture to remaining milk mixture in saucepan. Cook over low heat 1 minute longer. Remove from heat. Stir in softened gelatin. Pour 1 cup of hot mixture into a small bowl. Add chocolate and vanilla. Stir until blended. Pour into baked pie shell. Stir rum into remaining gelatin mixture. In a small bowl, beat egg whites until foamy; gradually add 1/3 cup sugar. Beat until stiff peaks form. Fold into rum mixture. Pour over chocolate layer in pie shell. Refrigerate until set. If desired, garnish with whipped cream and grated chocolate. Makes one 9-inch pie.

How To Make Black Bottom Pie

1/As the name indicates, this pie has a chocolate bottom and light top. To make this combination, add pre-melted chocolate to half the filling, then pour it into the bottom of the baked pie shell.

2/To make the light filling, add flavoring and sweetened stiffly beaten egg whites into remaining filling. Then spread over chocolate layer.

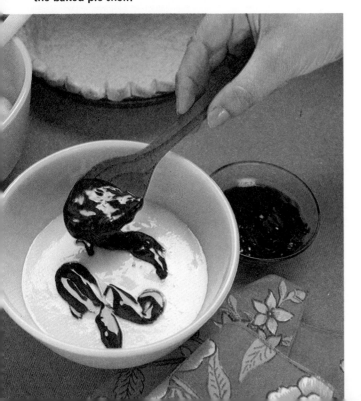

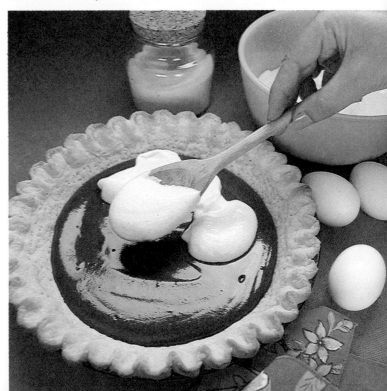

Nutty Pie Crust

Fill with your favorite chiffon or cream pie filling.

1 cup walnuts or almonds
2 oz. semisweet chocolate
2 tablespoons butter or margarine

2 tablespoons milk
3/4 cup sifted powdered sugar

Place nuts in blender container. Blend until finely chopped; set aside. Lightly grease a 9-inch pie pan; set aside. In a medium saucepan, combine chocolate, butter or margarine and milk. Stir constantly over low heat until chocolate melts. Remove from heat. Stir in powdered sugar and chopped nuts. Press on bottom and side of prepared pie pan. Refrigerate until set. Makes one 9-inch pie shell.

Cocoa Pie Crust

Chocolate crust sets off your favorite ice cream or pie filling.

1-1/4 cups flour
1/3 cup sugar
1/4 cup unsweetened cocoa powder
1/2 teaspoon salt

1/2 cup shortening
1/2 teaspoon vanilla extract
2 to 3 tablespoons cold water

Preheat oven to 400°F (205°C). In a medium bowl, combine flour, sugar, cocoa and salt. Cut in shortening with a pastry blender or 2 knives until pieces are size of small peas. Pour in vanilla and cold water. Mix until dough holds together. On a lightly floured board, roll out 1/8 inch thick. Place in a 9-inch pie pan. Trim and crimp edges. Bake 8 minutes. Pie crust will be soft and bubbly but will become firmer as it cools. Makes one 9-inch pie shell.

Coconut Nests

A different kind of tart crust for pudding, ice cream or pie filling.

4 oz. sweet cooking chocolate,
  broken in chunks

2 tablespoons butter or margarine
2 cups flaked coconut

Draw five 3-inch circles on wax paper. Place on a cookie sheet; set aside. Place chocolate and butter or margarine in a small saucepan. Stir constantly over low heat until chocolate melts. Remove from heat. Stir in coconut. Drop about 1/3 cup of coconut mixture on each circle and spread to cover circle. With back of a small spoon, scoop out centers and build up sides to form nests. Refrigerate until firm. Makes 5 nests.

Frozen Desserts

Chocolate-flavored frozen desserts have always been popular. In most cases they are easy to make and contain ingredients that are readily available. A great advantage to homemade frozen desserts is the fact that you can ensure the freshness and purity of the ingredients. You can eliminate chemical emulsifiers, stabilizers and artificial flavors found in most commercial products.

Another asset to making frozen desserts is that they can be made ahead, stored in the freezer and enjoyed anytime. If you plan to store a dessert for an extended period of time, especially in a so-called *frost-free* freezer, it should be tightly sealed to prevent icing and loss of moisture.

Chocolate Ice Cream

Make old-fashioned ice cream in your ice cream maker.

2 cups light cream
1/2 cup sugar
1 (6-oz.) pkg. semisweet chocolate pieces
   (1 cup)
3 egg yolks, slightly beaten

2 teaspoons vanilla extract
1 cup whipping cream (1/2 pint)
3 egg whites
1/2 cup sugar

In a medium saucepan, combine light cream, 1/2 cup sugar and chocolate pieces. Stir constantly over low heat until chocolate melts. Remove from heat. Stir about 1 cup chocolate mixture into beaten egg yolks. Add egg yolk mixture to remaining chocolate mixture in saucepan. Cook 2 or 3 minutes or until mixture begins to simmer. Remove from heat. Cool. Stir in vanilla and whipping cream. In a medium mixing bowl, beat egg whites until foamy. Gradually add 1/2 cup sugar. Beat until stiff. Fold cooled chocolate mixture into egg white mixture. Pour into liner of ice cream freezer and freeze according to manufacturer's directions. Makes 2 quarts.

Milk Chocolate Ice Cream

Smooth and creamy ice cream from the freezer of your refrigerator.

1 cup sugar
1 tablespoon cornstarch
3 cups milk
3 egg yolks, slightly beaten

1 teaspoon vanilla extract
1 cup milk chocolate pieces
3 egg whites
1 cup whipping cream (1/2 pint)

In a medium saucepan, combine sugar and cornstarch. Stir in milk. Stir constantly over medium heat until slightly thickened and smooth. Remove from heat. Mix about 1 cup hot mixture into beaten egg yolks. Add egg yolk mixture to remaining hot mixture in saucepan. Cook over low heat 3 minutes longer. Remove from heat. Add vanilla and milk chocolate pieces. Stir until chocolate melts. Cool. In a medium bowl, beat egg whites until stiff but not dry. Fold into cooled chocolate mixture. Spoon into a large mixer bowl. Freeze until almost frozen. Beat cream until stiff. Remove almost frozen chocolate mixture from freezer. Working quickly so mixture will not thaw completely, beat until fluffy. Fold in whipped cream. Immediately place in freezer. Freeze overnight or until firm. Makes about 1-3/4 quarts.

Mocha Chip Ice Cream

Chocolate flecks appear like magic when you add hot melted chocolate to the cold cream mixture.

1 cup sugar
1 tablespoon cornstarch
1 tablespoon instant coffee powder
1/8 teaspoon salt
2 cups light cream

6 eggs, slightly beaten
2 cups light cream
1 tablespoon vanilla extract
2 oz. semisweet chocolate

In a medium saucepan, combine sugar, cornstarch, coffee powder and salt. Stir in 2 cups cream. Stir constantly over low heat until thickened and bubbly. Stir about 1 cup hot mixture into beaten eggs. Add egg mixture to remaining hot mixture in saucepan. Cook and stir 1 minute longer. Chill. Stir in 2 cups cream and the vanilla. Melt chocolate. While chocolate is hot, pour it very slowly into chilled cream mixture, stirring constantly. Pour into liner of ice cream freezer. Freeze according to manufacturer's directions. Makes about 2 quarts.

How To Make Mocha Chip Ice Cream

1/Pour *hot* melted chocolate into *chilled* custard mixture. While pouring, stir custard mixture constantly to create miniature chocolate flecks.

2/Follow the freezer manufacturer's directions for proportions of salt and ice.

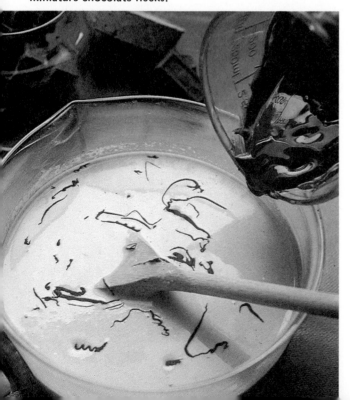

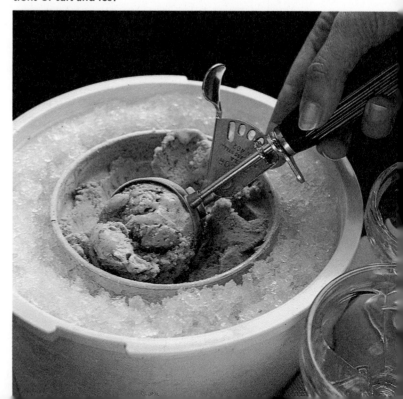

Butter Mint Ice Cream

Crushed mints and whipping cream add the final exquisite touch.

3 oz. semisweet chocolate
1-1/2 cups sugar
2 teaspoons cornstarch
2 cups light cream
1 cup milk

1/8 teaspoon salt
4 egg yolks, well-beaten
1/2 cup finely chopped butter mints
1 cup whipping cream

Melt chocolate; set aside; In a medium saucepan, combine sugar and cornstarch. Stir in light cream, milk and salt. Stir constantly over medium heat until mixture thickens. Remove from heat. Stir about 1 cup hot mixture into beaten egg yolks Add egg yolk mixture to remaining hot mixture in saucepan. Continue cooking over low heat 3 minutes. Stir in melted chocolate. Cool. Add crushed mints and whipping cream. Pour into liner of ice cream freezer. Freeze according to manufacturer's directions. Makes about 2 quarts.

Ice Cream Italiano

So smooth and rich because it's made with a base of Italian-style meringue.

1 cup milk
6 oz. semisweet chocolate
1 cup sugar
1/3 cup water

3 egg whites
1/4 teaspoon cream of tartar
1 cup whipping cream (1/2 pint)

In a small saucepan, heat milk and chocolate, stirring until chocolate melts. Simmer several minutes until mixture is the consistency of heavy cream. Set pan in ice. Stir until cool; set aside. In another small saucepan, bring sugar and water to a boil. Continue boiling without stirring until syrup reaches soft-ball stage or 238°F (115°C) on a candy thermometer. While sugar and water are boiling, beat egg whites in a large mixer bowl until foamy. Add cream of tartar; continue beating until stiff peaks form. Gradually pour syrup, which has reached soft-ball stage, into egg whites. Continue beating about 5 minutes or until cool. Fold in chocolate mixture. Whip cream; fold into chocolate mixture. Spoon into a plastic container, a bowl or ice trays. Cover. Freeze until firm. Makes about 2 quarts.

Alaska Pie

Lots of elegance with little effort!

1 cup chocolate cookie crumbs
  (13 to 15 cookies)
1/4 cup butter or margarine, melted
1 qt. peppermint or coffee ice cream,
  slightly softened

3 egg whites
1 cup marshmallow creme
Royal Chocolate Sauce, page 36

In a small bowl, combine cookie crumbs and melted butter or margarine. Press on bottom and sides of a 9-inch pie pan. Refrigerate until firm. Spoon ice cream over chocolate crust. Freeze. Preheat oven to 450°F (230°C). In a small mixer bowl, beat egg whites until stiff peaks form. Beat in marshmallow creme 1/4 cup at a time. Spoon onto frozen pie. Spread carefully, sealing to edge of crust. Bake 2 to 3 minutes or until golden. Serve immediately or return to freezer several hours or overnight. Serve with chocolate sauce. Makes 6 to 8 servings.

Ice Cream Meringue Pie

Like a chocolate sundae with crunch!

2 egg whites
1/2 cup sugar
1/2 teaspoon baking powder
1/4 teaspoon salt
1/2 cup graham cracker crumbs
  (7 crackers)

1/2 cup semisweet chocolate pieces
1 qt. butter pecan or black walnut ice cream
1/3 cup Royal Chocolate Sauce, page 36
  or Hot Fudge Sauce, page 37

Grease and flour a 9-inch pie pan; set aside. Preheat oven to 350°F (175°C). In a small mixer bowl, beat egg whites until frothy. Gradually add sugar. Beat until stiff and glossy. Fold in baking powder, salt, crumbs and chocolate pieces. Spoon into prepared pan, gently building up side with back of spoon. Bake 20 to 25 minutes. Cool. Fill with ice cream. Spoon chocolate syrup or fudge sauce over. Cut into wedges and serve immediately. Makes 6 to 8 servings.

A loaf pan is an excellent container for freezing ice cream.

Frozen Bananas

With a few bananas and wooden skewers you can relive a childhood pleasure!

1/4 cup butter or margarine
1 (6-oz.) pkg. semisweet chocolate pieces
   (1 cup)
3 tablespoons evaporated milk

6 or 7 bananas
1/3 cup finely chopped nuts, if desired

Line a cookie sheet with wax paper; set aside. In a 7- or 8-inch skillet over low heat and stirring constantly, melt butter or margarine and chocolate pieces. Stir in evaporated milk. Remove from heat. Peel bananas. Insert skewer into one end of each banana. Dip bananas 1 at a time into hot chocolate mixture, turning to coat completely. If desired, dip into chopped nuts before chocolate sets. Place on prepared cookie sheet; freeze. If not served the same day, freeze coated bananas in sealed freezer bags or wrap in aluminum foil. For a better eating consistency, remove from freezer 10 minutes before serving. Makes 6 or 7 chocolate-covered bananas.

Frozen Fudgies

Make sure you have paper cups and wooden skewers on hand.

1 (4-1/2-oz.) pkg. instant chocolate
   pudding mix

3-1/2 cups cold milk
1/4 cup sugar

In a medium mixing bowl, combine pudding mix with milk and sugar. Beat slowly 2 minutes with a rotary beater or electric mixer. Pour into eight 5-ounce paper cups. Freeze 1-1/2 to 2 hours or until partially frozen. Insert a wooden skewer into each. Freeze until firm. Peel off paper cups before serving. Makes 8 fudge bars.

Frozen Mint Cups

Cool and refreshing.

4 oz. unsweetened chocolate
1 cup butter, room temperature
2 cups powdered sugar

4 eggs
1/2 teaspoon peppermint extract

Line 8 custard cups with paper baking cups; set aside. Melt chocolate; set aside. In a large mixing bowl, cream butter and powdered sugar until light and fluffy. Add eggs 1 at a time, beating after each addition. Stir in melted chocolate and peppermint extract. Pour into lined custard cups. Freeze several hours. Just before serving, unmold onto serving plates. Makes 8 servings.

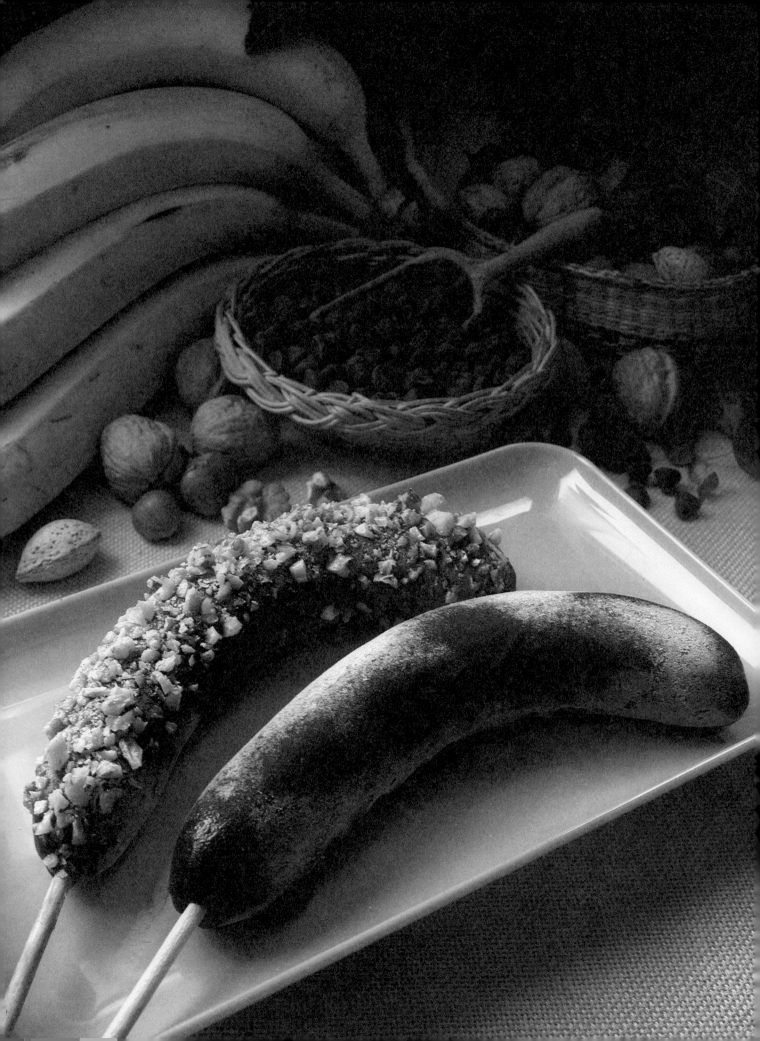

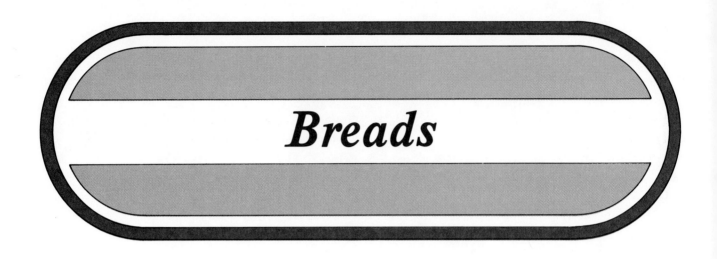

Breads

We all take great pride in preparing hot-from-the-oven treats for our family and friends. And the fragrance of home-baked chocolate bread is the most enticing of all!

Muffins are probably the fastest and easiest bread for a spur-of-the-moment baking spree. Choose basic Cocoa Muffins, Cinnamon Muffins or fantastic Banana-Bran Muffins with a delicate chocolate flavor. Make them in your regular muffin pans. Either grease the muffin cups and spoon the batter directly in, or line the muffin cups with fluted paper baking cups and pour batter into them.

Our favorite in this section is Sour Cream Coffee-cake. It has a rich cake-like appearance with a cocoa-cinnamon mixture swirled through the middle and over the top. We serve it warm on special occasions such as Christmas morning. It can be made ahead and frozen, then thawed and warmed just before serving. If you make Sour Cream Coffee-cake for the holidays, garnish it with cherries and chocolate leaves, see page 10, then lightly sift powdered sugar over the top for a snowy effect.

More time consuming, but just as rewarding, are the chocolate-flavored yeast breads. Start them 2 or 3 hours before you plan to serve them. Or make them a day ahead and reheat them just before serving.

For a special treat, try Cinnamon Waffles with butter and honey for brunch -- or topped with ice cream for dessert!

Frosted Chocolate Doughnuts

A tantalizing double-chocolate flavor.

1 egg
1/2 cup sugar
1 oz. unsweetened chocolate
1 tablespoon butter or margarine
1/2 cup mashed potatoes
1-3/4 cups flour

3 teaspoons baking powder
1/2 teaspoon salt
1/3 cup milk
Oil or shortening for frying
Chocolate Frosting, see below

Chocolate Frosting:
2 tablespoons butter or margarine
1 oz. unsweetened chocolate
1 cup sifted powdered sugar

2 tablespoons boiling water
1/4 teaspoon vanilla extract

In a large mixer bowl, beat egg until light. Beat in sugar. Melt chocolate and butter or margarine together. Add to egg mixture. Stir in potatoes. Combine flour, baking powder and salt. Add milk alternately with flour mixture. Refrigerate 1 hour. Preheat oil or shortening in deep-fryer or mini deep-fryer according to manufacturer's directions. On a lightly floured surface, roll out dough about 3/8 inch thick. Cut with floured doughnut cutter. Fry in hot oil or shortening about 2 minutes or until crusty brown. Drain and cool. Prepare Chocolate Frosting. Spread on doughnuts. Makes 12 to 14 doughnuts.

Chocolate Frosting:
In a medium saucepan, melt butter or margarine and chocolate. Beat in powdered sugar, boiling water and vanilla. Mix well.

Banana-Bran Muffins

Great taste and good for you.

1/4 cup butter or margarine
1/2 cup sugar
3 eggs
2 cups whole-bran cereal
1/2 cup buttermilk
1 cup flour

1 teaspoon salt
1-1/2 teaspoons baking soda
1/4 teaspoon ground allspice
2 tablespoons unsweetened cocoa powder
1-1/2 cups mashed ripe bananas
    (about 3 medium)

Grease 18 muffin cups; set aside. Preheat oven to 375°F (190°C). In a large mixer bowl, cream butter or margarine and sugar. Beat in eggs 1 at a time. Add cereal and buttermilk. Stir in flour, salt, baking soda, allspice and cocoa. Fold in bananas. Spoon into prepared muffin cups, filling each 2/3 full. Bake 15 minutes. Serve warm. Makes 18 muffins.

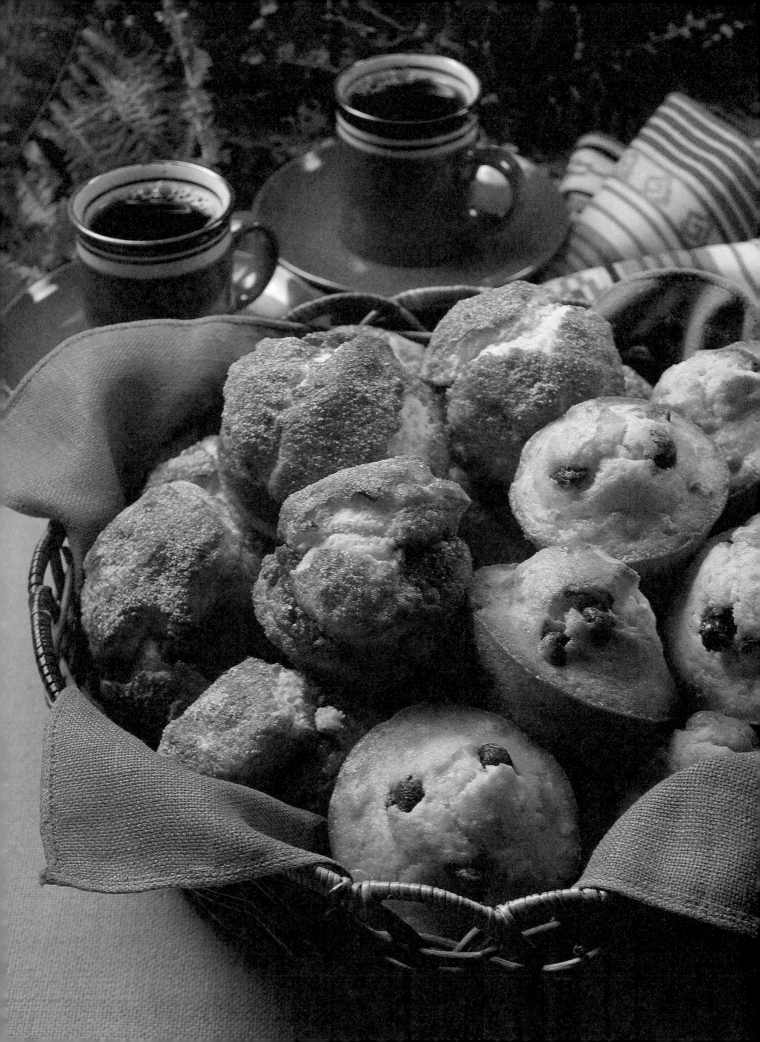

Cinnamon Muffins

Contrasting colors in a moist muffin.

2 cups flour
4 teaspoons baking powder
1/2 teaspoon salt
2 tablespoons sugar
2 eggs, slightly beaten
1 cup milk

1/4 cup butter, melted
1/4 cup sugar
1/2 teaspoon cinnamon
1 tablespoon sweetened chocolate-flavored
  instant cocoa mix

Grease 12 muffin cups; set aside. Preheat oven to 425°F (220°C). In a medium bowl, combine flour, baking powder, salt and 2 tablespoons sugar. In a small bowl, mix eggs, milk and melted butter. Stir egg mixture into flour mixture. Combine 1/4 cup sugar, cinnamon and cocoa mix. Spoon half of batter into prepared muffin cups. Sprinkle half of cinnamon-cocoa mixture over batter in cups. Spoon remaining batter on top. Sprinkle with remaining cinnamon-cocoa mixture. Bake 15 to 20 minutes or until golden brown. Serve hot. Makes 12 muffins.

Banana-Chip Muffins

Almost like a cake!

1-1/2 cups flour
1/2 cup sugar
2 teaspoons baking powder
1/2 teaspoon salt
1 egg, slightly beaten

1/2 cup milk
1/4 cup cooking oil
3/4 cup mashed ripe banana (about 2 small)
1/2 cup semisweet chocolate pieces
1/2 cup chopped walnuts

Grease 16 muffin cups; set aside. Preheat oven to 400°F (205°C). In a large bowl, combine flour, sugar, baking powder and salt. Add egg, milk, oil and bananas; stir until just combined. Stir in chocolate pieces and walnuts. Spoon into prepared muffin cups, filling each 2/3 full. Bake 20 to 25 minutes. Serve warm. Makes 16 muffins.

Cocoa Muffins

Good for breakfast or with a luncheon salad.

1 egg
1/2 cup milk
1/3 cup cooking oil
1-1/2 cups flour

1/2 cup sugar
3 tablespoons unsweetened cocoa powder
2 teaspoons baking powder
1/4 teaspoon salt

Grease 12 muffin cups; set aside. Preheat oven to 400°F (205°C). In a medium mixing bowl, beat egg. Stir in milk and oil. Add flour, sugar, cocoa, baking powder and salt; stir until flour is just moistened. Batter will be slightly lumpy. Fill prepared muffin cups 2/3 full. Bake 20 to 25 minutes. Makes 12 muffins.

From left to right: Cinnamon Muffins and Banana-Chip Muffins

Sour Cream Coffeecake

Terrific for brunch or snacks.

1/2 cup chopped nuts
1 teaspoon cinnamon
2 tablespoons sugar
1 tablespoon unsweetened cocoa powder
3/4 cup butter or margarine,
  room temperature
1-1/2 cups sugar

2 eggs
1 teaspoon vanilla extract
2-1/4 cups flour
2 teaspoons baking powder
1/2 teaspoon baking soda
1/2 teaspoon salt
1 cup dairy sour cream

Grease and flour a 10-inch tube pan; set aside. Preheat oven to 350°F (175°C). In a small bowl, combine nuts, cinnamon, 2 tablespoons sugar and the cocoa; set aside. In a large mixer bowl, cream butter or margarine and 1-1/2 cups sugar. Add eggs and vanilla, beating until light and fluffy. Combine flour, baking powder, baking soda and salt. Add flour mixture to creamed mixture in three portions, alternating with sour cream; beat well after each addition. Spread half of batter in prepared pan. Sprinkle with half of cinnamon-nut mixture. Spoon in remaining batter and sprinkle with remaining cinnamon-nut mixture. Bake 45 to 50 minutes. Cool in pan 15 minutes. Remove from pan and serve warm or cool. Makes one 10-inch tube cake.

Pull-Apart Ring

Enjoy this new version of Monkey Bread.

1 (13-3/4-oz.) pkg. hot roll mix
3/4 cup very warm water, 105°F to 115°F
  (40°C to 45°C)
2 tablespoons sugar
1 egg

1/2 cup sugar
1/2 teaspoon cinnamon
1 tablespoon unsweetened cocoa powder
1/3 cup finely chopped nuts
1/3 cup butter or margarine, melted

In a large bowl, dissolve yeast from hot roll mix in warm water. Stir in 2 tablespoons sugar and the egg. Add flour mixture from hot roll mix. Blend well. Cover. Let rise in a warm place until doubled in bulk, 30 to 45 minutes. Grease a 10-inch tube pan; set aside. In a small bowl, combine 1/2 cup sugar, cinnamon, cocoa and nuts; set aside. On a floured surface, shape dough into a round ball, working in a small amount of flour from the floured surface if dough is sticky. Cut into 24 pieces. Dip each piece into melted butter, then into cocoa-nut mixture. Arrange pieces about 1/4 inch apart in layers in prepared pan. Cover. Let rise again until doubled in bulk, 20 to 40 minutes. Preheat oven to 375°F (190°C). Bake 30 to 35 minutes or until golden brown. Cool in pan 2 minutes. Invert on serving plate; remove pan. Serve warm. Makes 24 pieces.

Sticky Buns

Sticky and gooey, but really good.

1 (13-3/4-oz.) pkg. hot roll mix
Liquid according to pkg. directions
Egg according to pkg. directions
1/2 cup butter or margarine
1 cup light brown sugar, lightly packed
1/2 cup light corn syrup

2 tablespoons butter or margarine, melted
1/2 cup chopped pecans
1/2 cup light brown sugar, lightly packed
1 teaspoon cinnamon
1/2 cup semisweet chocolate pieces

Prepare hot roll mix according to package directions. Cover; let rise in a warm place until doubled in bulk. Grease two 8-inch cake pans; set aside. In a small saucepan, melt 1/2 cup butter or margarine. Stir in 1 cup brown sugar and the corn syrup. Cook over low heat until sugar dissolves. Pour half of syrupy mixture into each prepared pan. Roll out dough on a floured surface to a 14" x 9" rectangle. Brush rectangle with 2 tablespoons melted butter or margarine. Combine pecans, 1/2 cup brown sugar, the cinnamon and chocolate pieces. Sprinkle over buttered dough. Starting with longer edge, roll up dough jelly-roll style; press edge to seal. Cut into sixteen 7/8-inch slices. Place 8 slices in each cake pan, cut side down in syrup. Cover. Let rise in a warm place until doubled in bulk. Preheat oven to 350°F (175°C). Bake 20 to 25 minutes or until golden brown. Cool in pan about 5 minutes. Invert on serving plate; remove pan. Serve warm. Makes 16 buns.

How To Make Sticky Buns

1/ Sprinkle pecans, brown sugar, cinnamon and chocolate pieces to within about 1/2 inch of edges of dough rectangle. Starting with longer edge of dough, carefully roll up jelly-roll style.

2/With a sharp knife, cut roll into 16 pinwheel slices. With a spatula, place 8 slices on top of the syrupy mixture in each pan. Cover and let rise in warm place before baking.

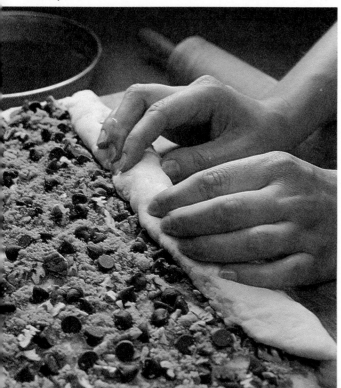

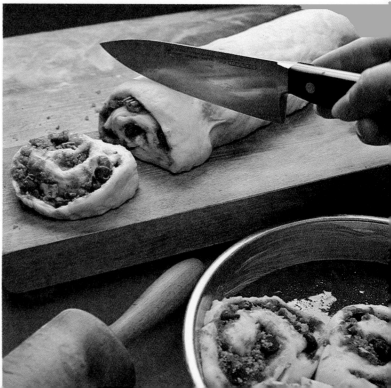

Spicy Chocolate Loaf
Moist, spicy and delicious!

2 oz. semisweet chocolate	1/3 cup shortening
1-1/2 cups flour	2 eggs
1 cup sugar	1/2 cup applesauce
1 teaspoon baking soda	1/4 teaspoon nutmeg
1/4 teaspoon baking powder	1/2 teaspoon cinnamon
1/2 teaspoon salt	1/3 cup chopped nuts

Melt chocolate; set aside. Grease and flour a 9" x 5" loaf pan; set aside. Preheat oven to 350°F (175°C). In a large mixer bowl, combine all ingredients except chocolate and nuts. Beat 3 minutes with electric mixer on medium speed. Stir in melted chocolate and nuts. Pour into prepared pan. Bake 50 to 55 minutes. Remove from pan; cool thoroughly before slicing. Makes 1 loaf.

Festive Holiday Bread
Here's the recipe you've been waiting for!

1 cup orange juice	1 egg
1 cup milk	1 (6-oz.) pkg. semisweet chocolate pieces
1/4 cup cooking oil	(1cup)
2 cups flour	1 cup chopped candied fruits
1/2 cup sugar	1 teaspoon grated orange peel
1 tablespoon salt	About 2-1/2 cups flour
2 pkgs. active dry yeast	Citrus Glaze, see below.

Citrus Glaze:

1 cup powdered sugar	2 tablespoons orange juice
1 tablespoon butter or margarine, melted	

In a small saucepan, heat orange juice, milk and oil until very warm (120° to 130°F, 50° to 55°C). In a large mixer bowl, combine 2 cups flour, the sugar, salt and yeast. Add warm milk mixture and egg. Beat at low speed until moistened, then medium speed 3 minutes. Stir in chocolate pieces, candied fruits, orange peel and enough flour to form a stiff batter. Cover. Let rise in a warm place until doubled in bulk, 45 to 60 minutes. Generously grease a 10-inch fluted tube pan; set aside. Preheat oven to 350°F (175°C). Stir down batter. Spoon into prepared pan. Bake 40 to 50 minutes or until golden brown. Immediately remove from pan. Cool slightly. Prepare Citrus Glaze. Spoon glaze over bread, letting excess drip down sides. Makes one 10-inch tube bread.

Citrus Glaze:
Combine all ingredients in a small bowl; mix well.

Cinnamon Waffles

An impressive and tasty dessert with very little effort.

2 egg yolks
1/4 cup butter or margarine, melted
1 cup dairy sour cream
1 cup buttermilk
1 cup flour
1/4 cup sugar
1 teaspoon baking soda

1/4 teaspoon salt
1/2 teaspoon cinnamon
2 tablespoons unsweetened cocoa powder
2 egg whites
Powdered sugar
1 (16-oz.) can cherry or peach pie filling

In a large mixer bowl, beat egg yolks until thickened and lemon-colored. Add melted butter or margarine, sour cream and buttermilk. Beat until blended. Add flour, sugar, baking soda, salt, cinnamon and cocoa. Beat until smooth. Preheat waffle iron. In a small mixer bowl, beat egg whites until stiff but not dry. Fold into cocoa batter. Spoon on preheated waffle iron. Close lid and bake until brown and crisp. Remove from waffle iron. Repeat until all batter is used. Sprinkle waffles with powdered sugar. Top with pie filling. Makes 8 or 9 waffles.

Brownie Waffles

Rich and brownie-like with a tantalizing aroma while baking.

1 (6-oz.) pkg. semisweet chocolate pieces
   (1 cup)
3/4 cup milk
1/2 cup butter or margarine
2 egg yolks
1/3 cup sugar

1-1/2 cups flour
1/2 teaspoon baking powder
1/4 teaspoon salt
1/4 cup chopped nuts
2 egg whites
Ice cream

In a small saucepan over low heat, heat chocolate pieces, milk and butter or margarine until chocolate pieces melt. Remove from heat; set aside. Preheat waffle iron. In a large mixer bowl, beat egg yolks until thickened and lemon-colored. Gradually beat in sugar. Add melted chocolate mixture, then flour, baking powder and salt. Mix well. Stir in nuts. In a small mixer bowl, beat egg whites until stiff but not dry. Fold into chocolate batter. Spoon on preheated waffle iron. Close lid and bake until crisp. Remove from waffle iron. Repeat until all batter is used. Top with your favorite ice cream. Makes about 6 waffles.

Beverages

There are almost as many products for making chocolate drinks as there are ways to do it. For a quick glass of chocolate milk or a cup of hot cocoa in the morning before school or work, it's handy to have one of the instant chocolate mixes on hand. Some of these are available in individual packets where the mix is pre-measured. Others are sold in 1/2-pound or 1-pound containers and you measure the amount needed. Suggested amounts are given in the directions on the container.

We have included recipes for making traditional Hot Cocoa or Hot Chocolate. Try them to see which you like best. For a special-occasion breakfast, French Chocolate is a memorable treat.

Chocolate is an ideal flavor partner with many liqueurs for creating interesting, unconventional after-dinner drinks. They can even take the place of desserts! Your guests will be impressed with your originality and you'll be pleased with the elegant effect and so little work.

Hot Cocoa

The blend of cocoa and milk produces a very appealing beverage.

3 tablespoons unsweetened cocoa powder
1/4 cup sugar

2 cups milk
Marshmallows, if desired

In a small saucepan, combine cocoa and sugar. Pour in about 1/4 cup of milk, stirring to form a smooth paste. Gradually stir in remaining milk. Heat over low heat but do not boil. Remove from heat. Beat until foamy. Pour into 3 cups. Top each with a marshmallow, if desired. Makes 3 servings.

Hot Chocolate

Something to anticipate on a cold day.

1 oz. unsweetened chocolate
2 tablespoons water
1/4 cup sugar

2 cups milk
1/4 teaspoon vanilla extract

In a small saucepan, combine chocolate and water. Stir over very low heat until chocolate melts. Add sugar. Stir until blended. Gradually stir in milk. Heat thoroughly, stirring occasionally. Makes 3 to 4 servings.

French Chocolate

Superbly elegant treat for eight or second servings for four.

2 oz. semisweet chocolate
1/4 cup light corn syrup
3 tablespoons water

1/2 teaspoon vanilla extract
1 cup whipping cream (1/2 pint)
4 cups milk

In a small saucepan, stir chocolate, corn syrup and water over low heat until chocolate melts and mixture is smooth. If a few flecks of chocolate remain, beat briefly with a whisk. Stir in vanilla. Chill. Beat cream until almost stiff. Add chilled chocolate mixture gradually, continuing to beat until mixture mounds when dropped from a spoon. Refrigerate. Just before serving, heat milk until very hot but not boiling. Spoon whipped cream mixture equally into 8 cups. Fill cups with hot milk; blend. Serve immediately. Makes 8 servings.

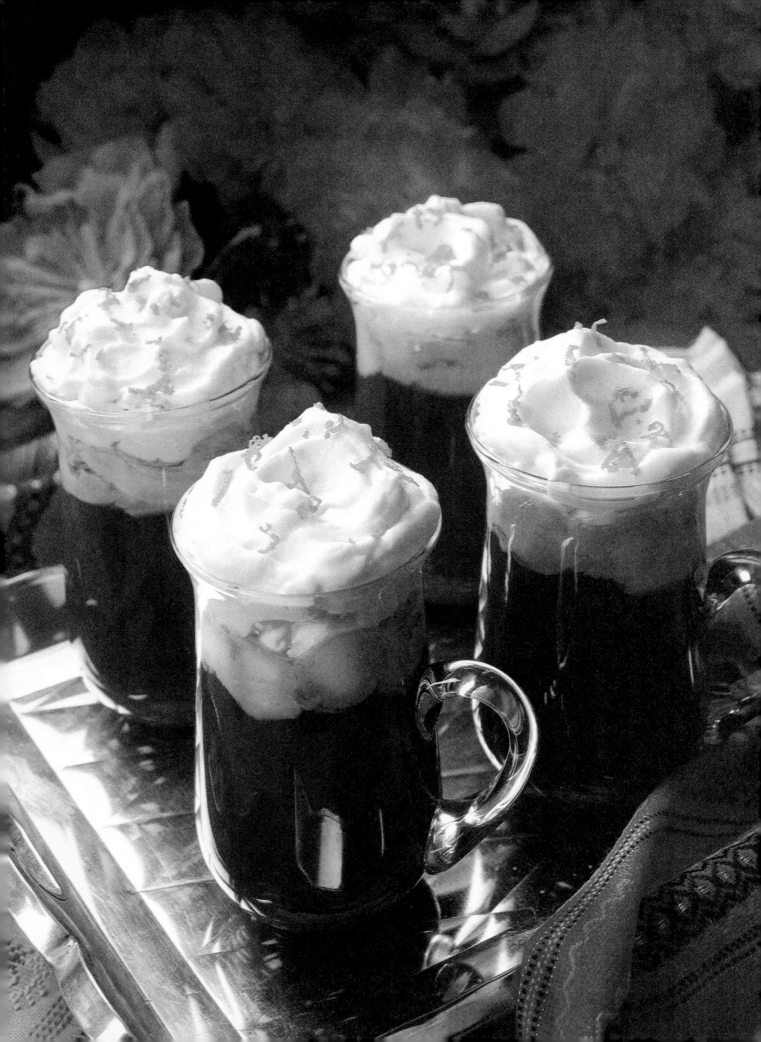

Cafe Bahia

A scrumptious after-dinner drink—or a dessert.

2 cups strong coffee
1/4 cup chocolate syrup
2 tablespoons brandy
2 tablespoons coffee-flavored liqueur
1/8 teaspoon nutmeg

1/2 cup whipping cream
2 tablespoons orange-flavored liqueur
Grated sweet chocolate or
   grated orange peel

In a small saucepan, heat coffee, chocolate syrup, brandy, coffee liqueur and nutmeg. While coffee mixture is heating, whip cream until stiff. Fold in orange liqueur. Pour hot coffee mixture into 4 mugs or heatproof glasses. Top with whipped cream, then grated chocolate or orange peel. Makes 4 servings.

Café au Lait

Try this on a cold night in front of a glowing fire.

2 cups strong coffee
2 cups milk
1/4 cup chocolate syrup

1/2 cup whipping cream
2 tablespoons crème de cacao
Grated chocolate

In a medium saucepan, heat coffee, milk and chocolate syrup. Remove from heat. While coffee mixture is heating, whip cream. Fold in crème de cacao. Pour hot coffee mixture into 5 coffee cups or heatproof glasses. Top with whipped cream and grated chocolate. Makes 5 servings.

Old Amsterdam Coffee

This extravagantly flavored coffee can be a dessert too.

2 cups strong hot coffee
2 tablespoons white crème de menthe
2 tablespoons chocolate-mint liqueur

Whipped cream
Grated semisweet chocolate

Combine hot coffee with crème de menthe and chocolate-mint liqueur. Pour into 4 small cups or heatproof glasses. Top with whipped cream, then grated chocolate. Serve immediately. Makes 4 servings.

Grasshopper Frappé

Delightfully refreshing.

1 pint chocolate ice cream
1/4 cup white crème de menthe

1/4 cup crème de cacao
Chocolate curls, if desired

In blender container, combine ice cream with crème de menthe and crème de cacao. Blend until smooth. Pour into 4 small glasses. If desired, sprinkle with chocolate curls. Serve at once. Makes 4 drinks.

Banana Eggnog

Terrific as an after-school snack or a quick breakfast.

1 large banana, peeled
1 egg
3 tablespoons sweetened chocolate-flavored
  instant cocoa mix

2 cups cold milk

Break banana into 4 or 5 pieces. In blender container, combine banana, egg, cocoa mix and milk. Blend until smooth. Makes 2 servings.

Homemade Crème de Cacao

An excellent chocolate liqueur that is both thrifty and easy.

1 cup sugar
2 cups water
1 oz. unsweetened chocolate

1/2 teaspoon vanilla extract
1 cup vodka

In a medium saucepan, combine sugar and water. Boil on medium-high heat until mixture is reduced to half its volume, about 20 minutes. About 5 minutes before syrup is done, melt chocolate in a 2-cup or larger container. Immediately, very slowly pour hot syrup into the melted chocolate, stirring vigorously while pouring. If mixture is not completely smooth and blended, beat with mixer or in blender. Cool mixture 30 minutes. Add vanilla and vodka, blending well. Immediately pour into bottle or jar with tight fitting cap or lid. Makes about 1 pint liqueur.

Black & White Ice Cream Sodas

Purists may use chocolate ice cream instead of vanilla.

1/2 cup cold milk
1/4 cup chocolate syrup
4 scoops vanilla ice cream

Cold club soda
Whipped cream
2 maraschino cherries

Mix milk with chocolate syrup. Pour into 2 tall glasses. Add 1 scoop ice cream to each glass. Pour in a small amount of cold soda; mash ice cream in each glass with back of a long-handled spoon. Add second scoop of ice cream to each glass. Fill glasses with soda. Garnish with whipped cream and a cherry. Makes 2 servings.

How To Make Black & White Ice Cream Sodas

1/Mash ice cream in the glass with the back of a spoon to mix it with the other ingredients.

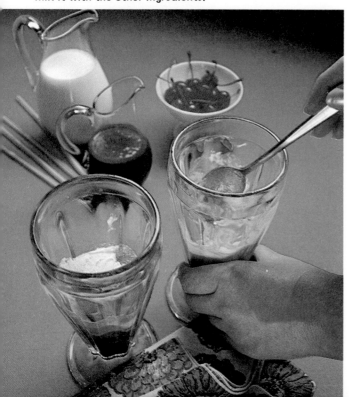

2/Top your sodas with a second scoop of ice cream. Fill the glasses with cold soda. To give an authentic touch, top with whipped cream and maraschino cherries.

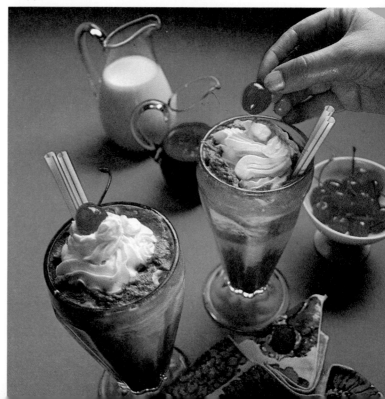

Potpourri

This is the section where you'll find an assortment of traditional chocolate dishes that have very little in common -- except chocolate.

Several variations of chocolate fondue will remind you of the fun of this party dish. We like to dip into Chocolate Fondue with cubes of angel-food or pound cake, marshmallows, pecan or walnut halves and all kinds of fresh fruits. The next time you entertain, round up your own favorite ingredients and bring out the fondue pot!

Bavarian Crepes are an impressive dessert, yet you can make the crepes ahead of time and avoid last minute confusion.

No one is able to resist Éclairs and Cream Puffs. They've always been among the most admired desserts in fancy bakeries and on pastry carts in elegant restaurants. As a variation of the puff family, you'll enjoy our classic Profiteroles with chocolate sauce. They are miniature cream puffs filled with ice cream or cream filling and topped with chocolate. Look for other ideas for fillings for Cream Puffs, Éclairs or crepes in Frostings, Fillings & Sauces, pages 30 to 40.

Éclairs

Everybody's favorite!

1/2 cup butter or margarine	4 eggs
1 cup water	Custard-Cream Filling, below
1 cup flour	Traditional Glaze, see below
1/4 teaspoon salt	

Traditional Glaze:

1 oz. unsweetened chocolate	1 cup sifted powdered sugar
1 teaspoon butter	2 tablespoons hot water

Lightly grease a cookie sheet; set aside. Preheat oven to 400°F (205°C). In a medium saucepan, heat butter or margarine and water to a rolling boil. Add flour and salt all at once. Stir vigorously over low heat about 1 minute or until mixture becomes smooth and does not cling to side of pan. Remove from heat. Beat in eggs 1 at a time. Beat until mixture no longer looks slippery. Assemble pastry bag with a plain round tip that has a 1/2- to 3/4-inch opening. Put mixture through pastry bag onto prepared cookie sheet, forming strips 1-1/2 inches thick and 4-1/2 inches long. Or use a small spoon to form strips of dough. Bake 30 to 40 minutes. Cool away from draft. Split cold éclairs. Fill each éclair with 3 to 4 tablespoons Custard-Cream Filling. Prepare Traditional Glaze. Spoon over filled éclairs, letting excess drip down sides. Refrigerate until serving time. Makes 10 éclairs.

Traditional Glaze:

In a small saucepan, melt chocolate and butter over low heat. Remove from heat. Stir in powdered sugar and water. Beat until smooth.

Custard-Cream Filling

The touch of perfection for Éclairs, above, or Cream Puffs, page 144.

1/3 cup sugar	1-1/2 cups milk
1 tablespoon flour	1 egg yolk, slightly beaten
1 tablespoon cornstarch	1 teaspoon vanilla extract
1/4 teaspoon salt	1/2 cup whipping cream

In a medium saucepan, combine sugar, flour, cornstarch and salt. Gradually stir in milk. Stir constantly over medium heat until mixture boils and thickens. Remove from heat. Stir a small amount of hot milk mixture into egg yolk. Add egg yolk mixture to remaining hot milk mixture in saucepan. Stir over low heat another 2 minutes. Stir in vanilla. Cover surface with plastic wrap. Cool. Whip cream; fold into cool custard. Makes enough to fill 10 Éclairs or 9 Cream Puffs.

Yule Log

Our version of the traditional Bûche Noël is time-consuming but worth it!

5 egg yolks	3/4 teaspoon baking powder
2/3 cup sugar	1/4 teaspoon salt
1/2 teaspoon vanilla extract	Powdered sugar
5 egg whites	Buttercream Filling, see below
1/2 cup sugar	Meringue Mushrooms, page 106
1-1/2 cups sifted cake flour	

Buttercream Filling:

2 oz. unsweetened chocolate	3 egg yolks
1 cup sugar	1/2 cup butter, room temperature
1/2 cup water	1 tablespoon rum

Grease a 15" x 10" baking pan and line with wax paper. Grease wax paper; set aside. Grease 2 custard cups; set aside. Preheat oven to 375°F (190°C). In a small mixer bowl, beat egg yolks until thickened and lemon-colored, about 5 minutes. Gradually add 2/3 cup sugar, beating constantly. Stir in vanilla. In a large mixer bowl, beat egg whites until foamy. Gradually add 1/2 cup sugar, beating until stiff but not dry. Fold egg yolk mixture into beaten egg whites. Sift together flour, baking powder and salt. Fold into egg mixture. Spoon about 2 tablespoons batter into each prepared custard cup. Gently spread remaining batter in prepared pan. Bake 10 to 12 minutes. Sprinkle powdered sugar on a clean, dry dish towel. When cake is done, loosen edges and immediately invert on prepared towel. Remove pan and wax paper. Starting with longer edge of cake, roll up cake and towel together. Cool. Remove cake from custard cups; cool. Prepare Buttercream Filling. Unroll cake; remove towel. Spread cake with half of filling. Reroll cake without towel and frost with remaining filling. Lightly press both cakes from custard cups into filling along side of log to resemble knots. Spread filling over all. Swirl with a spatula or score with a fork to resemble bark. Slice and serve. Garnish with Meringue Mushrooms. Makes 10 to 12 servings.

Buttercream Filling:

Melt chocolate; set aside to cool. In a small saucepan, bring sugar and water to a boil. Cook to 240°F (115°C) on a candy thermometer or soft-ball stage. Remove from heat. While candy is cooking, beat egg yolks in a small mixer bowl until thickened and lemon-colored. Very gradually add hot syrup, beating constantly. Continue beating until lukewarm. Beat in butter 1 tablespoon at a time. Mix in melted chocolate and rum. Beat until thickened.

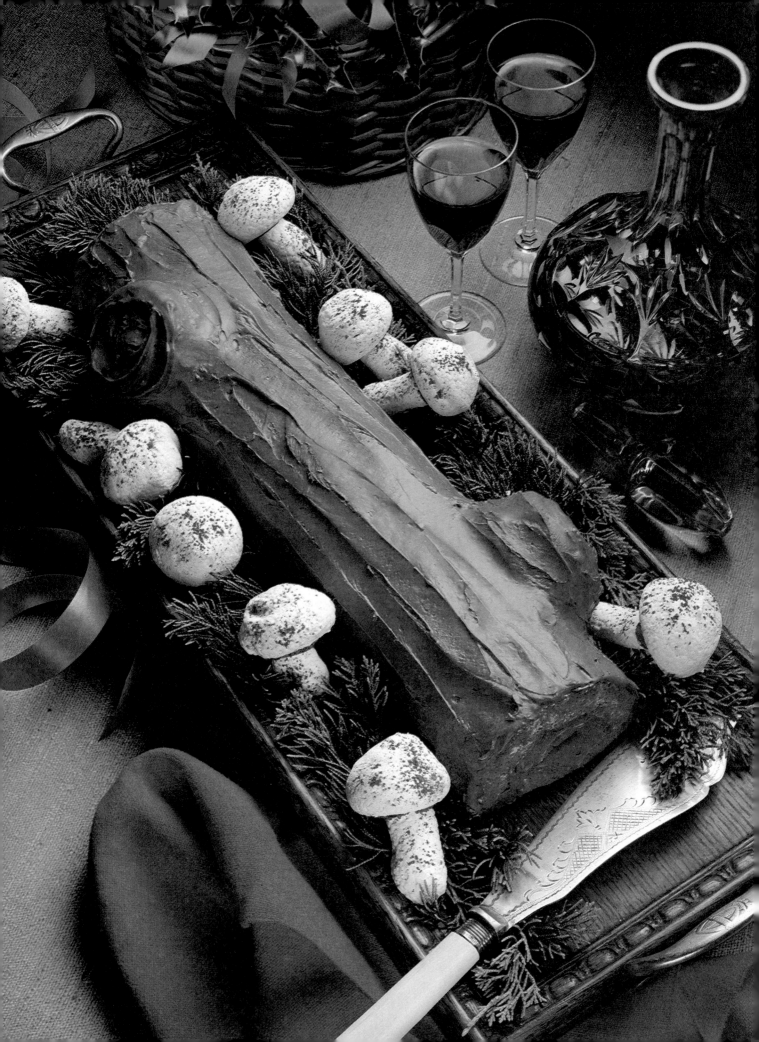

Cream Puffs

Even the cream puff shells are chocolate-flavored.

3/4 cup flour

1 tablespoon unsweetened cocoa powder

1 tablespoon sugar

1/8 teaspoon salt

1 cup water

1/2 cup butter or margarine

4 eggs

Custard-Cream Filling, page 141

Almond-Butter Glaze, see below

Almond-Butter Glaze:

2 oz. unsweetened chocolate

1/4 cup butter or margarine

1-1/2 cups sifted powdered sugar

1 tablespoon almond-flavored liqueur

2 tablespoons hot water

Grease cookie sheet; set aside. Preheat oven to 400°F (205°C). Stir together flour, cocoa, sugar and salt; set aside. In a medium saucepan, bring water and butter or margarine to a boil. Quickly stir in flour mixture over low heat, beating vigorously with a spoon until mixture forms a ball. Remove from heat. Add eggs 1 at a time, beating with a spoon after each addition until mixture is shiny and smooth. To make 9 puffs, spoon about 1/4 cup mixture for each puff onto prepared cookie sheet about 3 inches apart. Bake 35 to 45 minutes or until puffed and firm. Split in half while hot; cool. Fill each cooled puff with about 3 tablespoons Custard Cream Filling. Prepare Almond Glaze. Immediately spoon glaze over filled cream puffs, letting excess drip down sides. Refrigerate until serving time. Makes 9 cream puffs.

Almond-Butter Glaze:

In a small saucepan, melt chocolate and butter or margarine over low heat. Remove from heat. Stir in powdered sugar, liqueur and hot water. Continue stirring until smooth.

Make a double batch of crepes and freeze half of them for another recipe at a later time.

Profiteroles

Miniature cream puffs filled with ice cream and topped with rich dark chocolate.

1/4 cup butter or margarine	2 eggs
1/2 cup water	Dark Chocolate Sauce, see below
1/2 cup flour	1 pint vanilla or chocolate ice cream
1/8 teaspoon salt	

Dark Chocolate Sauce

2 oz. unsweetened chocolate, broken in small chunks	1/2 cup sugar
1/4 cup water	3 tablespoons butter or margarine
	1/2 teaspoon vanilla extract

Lightly grease cookie sheets; set aside. Preheat oven to 400°F (205°C). In a medium saucepan, heat butter or margarine and water to a rolling boil. Add flour and salt all at once. Stir vigorously over low heat about 1 minute or until mixture becomes smooth and does not cling to side of pan. Remove from heat. Beat in eggs 1 at a time. Beat until mixture no longer looks slippery. Drop from a teaspoon onto prepared cookie sheets forming 33 to 36 mounds about 3/4 inch across. Bake 10 to 15 minutes. Cool away from draft. Prepare Dark Chocolate Sauce. When puffs are cool, split in half. Place about 1 tablespoon ice cream inside each. Arrange in groups of 3 on individual dessert dishes. Drizzle tops with warm chocolate sauce. Serve immediately. Makes 11 to 12 servings.

Dark Chocolate Sauce:

In a small saucepan over low heat, combine chocolate, water and sugar, stirring constantly, until chocolate melts. Bring to a boil. Simmer 5 minutes or until slightly thickened. Remove from heat. Stir in butter or margarine and vanilla. Let cool slightly.

Peanut Butter Fondue

If you crave peanut butter with chocolate, you won't be able to stop dipping into this fondue.

1 (6-oz.) pkg. semisweet chocolate pieces (1 cup)	1/4 cup peanut butter
	Angel-food cake squares
1 (14-oz.) can sweetened condensed milk	Marshmallows
1 teaspoon vanilla extract	Banana slices
1/4 cup whole milk	Orange sections

In a medium saucepan, combine chocolate pieces, condensed milk, vanilla and whole milk. Stir constantly over low heat until chocolate melts. Stir in peanut butter. Pour into fondue pot; place over heat. With fondue forks or long skewers, dip cake squares, marshmallows or fruits into hot fondue. Makes about 2-1/3 cups fondue.

Chocolate Fondue

Get your fondue pot out of hiding and enjoy chocolate in a new way!

6 oz. unsweetened chocolate
1 cup light cream
1-1/2 cups sugar
1/2 cup butter or margarine
1/8 teaspoon salt
3 tablespoons crème de cacao
   or coffee-flavored liqueur

Angel-food cake squares
Whole strawberries
Banana slices
Orange sections

In a saucepan, melt chocolate in cream over very low heat. Stir in sugar, butter or margarine and salt. Stir constantly over very low heat until smooth. Stir in liqueur. Pour into fondue pot; place over heat. With fondue forks or long skewers, dip cake squares or fruits into sauce. Makes about 3 cups fondue.

Mocha Fondue

A serve-yourself dessert for your next dinner party.

1/2 cup butter or margarine
1 (12-oz.) pkg. semisweet chocolate pieces
   (2 cups)
6 tablespoons evaporated milk, not diluted
2 tablespoons instant coffee powder

Marshmallows
Chunks of pound cake
Banana chunks
Orange sections

In a medium saucepan over low heat, stirring constantly, melt butter or margarine and chocolate pieces. Stir in evaporated milk and coffee powder. Pour into fondue pot; place over heat. With fondue forks or long skewers, dip marshmallows, cake or fruits into fondue. Makes about 2-1/2 cups fondue.

Bavarian Crepes

Indescribably elegant and delicious!

2 eggs
1 cup buttermilk
3/4 cup flour
2 tablespoons sugar
2 tablespoons unsweetened cocoa powder

2 tablespoons butter, melted
Cherry Filling, see below
1 cup dairy sour cream
1 oz. semisweet chocolate, grated

Cherry Filling
2 (16-oz.) cans sweet, dark pitted cherries
1 cup powdered sugar
2 tablespoons cornstarch

1/2 cup almond-flavored liqueur
1 cup dairy sour cream
1 oz. semisweet chocolate, grated

In a medium bowl, beat eggs slightly. Add buttermilk. Beat with a whisk or with electric mixer on low speed until just blended. Add flour, sugar and cocoa, beating with whisk or with electric mixer on medium speed until smooth. Beat in melted butter. Let batter stand about 1/2 hour at room temperature. If kept longer before cooking, refrigerate. Stir batter with a spoon. Cook crepes on upside down crepe griddle or in traditional crepe or omelet pan. As each crepe is cooked, stack in a covered dish or pan to keep warm and moist. Prepare Cherry Filling. Spoon onto warm cooked crepes. Fold sides over filling, envelope-style. Spoon sour cream on top. Sprinkle with grated chocolate. Serve immediately. Makes 14 to 16 servings.

Cherry Filling

Drain cherries, reserving 1/3 cup juice. In a medium saucepan, combine powdered sugar and cornstarch. Stir in liqueur and reserved cherry juice. Add drained cherries. Stir constantly over moderate heat until slightly thickened.

Dark Chocolate Cups

Delectable chocolate cups filled with your favorite ice cream or pudding.

4 oz. semisweet chocolate
16 to 20 fluted paper or foil baking cups

Desired filling

Melt chocolate in top of double boiler over hot but not boiling water. Remove double boiler from heat but leave top part over hot water. Use a double thickness of paper or foil cups. Dip a new clean, dry 1/2-inch brush in melted chocolate. Brush on bottom and sides of cups 1/16 to 1/8 inch thick, pushing chocolate into ridges and smoothing as much as possible. Place in muffin pan cups. Chill until set. Carefully peel off paper or foil. Fill with desired filling. Makes 8 to 10 cups.

Variation

Light Chocolate Cups: Substitute 1/2 cup milk chocolate pieces and 1/2 cup semisweet chocolate pieces for 4 ounces semisweet chocolate. Use 20 to 24 baking cups. Makes 10 to 12 cups.

Roast Chicken Mole

Mole (moh-leh) is an unexpectedly tasty Mexican sauce made with unsweetened chocolate.

1 medium onion, chopped
1 garlic clove, minced
2 tablespoons cooking oil
2 tablespoons sugar
2 tablespoons flour
1 teaspoon salt
1/2 teaspoon cinnamon
1 teaspoon chili powder

1/2 teaspoon ground cumin
1/2 teaspoon oregano
1 (1-oz.) pkg. pre-melted unsweetened
  baking chocolate
1 (16-oz.) can tomatoes, cut up
1 cup chicken broth or bouillon
1 (4- to 5-lb.) roasting chicken

In a medium saucepan, sauté onion and garlic in oil until tender. In a small bowl, mix sugar, flour, salt, cinnamon, chili powder, cumin and oregano. Stir into onion mixture. Add chocolate, tomatoes and chicken broth or bouillon. Bring to a boil, stirring constantly. Simmer, stirring occasionally, 5 minutes. Remove giblets from chicken; pat chicken dry. Preheat oven to 350°F (175°C). Place chicken in roasting pan without a rack. Spoon sauce over chicken. Cover with aluminum foil. Roast 1-1/4 to 1-1/2 hours or until tender, basting several times with sauce. To serve, carve chicken; spoon sauce over all. Makes 5 to 6 servings.

Variation
Chicken may be cut up before roasting with sauce.

Pears Hélène

Glamorize this easy-to-make, classic dessert with whipped cream trim.

8 canned pear halves
1 oz. semisweet chocolate,
  broken in small chunks
1/4 cup water
1/4 cup sugar

1/4 cup light corn syrup
1 tablespoon butter or margarine
4 scoops vanilla ice cream
Whipped cream, if desired
Maraschino cherries, if desired

Refrigerate pears. Combine chocolate, water, sugar and corn syrup in a small saucepan. Stir constantly over low heat until chocolate melts. Remove from heat. Beat in butter or margarine. If sauce is not smooth, beat with a wire whisk or rotary beater. Set aside to cool about 5 minutes. Drain chilled pears. Place a scoop of ice cream in center of each of 4 pear halves. Top with remaining pear halves, forming 4 whole stuffed pears. Spoon about 2 tablespoons chocolate sauce into each of 4 dessert dishes. Stand one whole stuffed pear on end in chocolate sauce in each dessert dish. Spoon remaining chocolate sauce over each. If desired, pipe a ruffle of whipped cream around edges of pears where the halves come together. Top with a cherry, if desired. Makes 4 servings.

Variation
Use 4 whole fresh pears. Peel, halve and core pears. In a medium saucepan, combine 2 cups water and 1 cup sugar. Bring to a boil. Drop in pears and simmer until tender. Remove from heat; refrigerate in syrup. Proceed as directed.

Chantilly Lace Cones

Be prepared—have a few scraps of aluminum foil ready to prevent collapsed cones.

1/4 cup butter
1/4 cup light corn syrup
1/3 cup light brown sugar, lightly packed
2 teaspoons unsweetened cocoa powder
1/8 teaspoon cinnamon

1/2 cup flour
1/4 cup finely chopped nuts
3/4 pint whipping cream (1-1/2 cups)
3 tablespoons powdered sugar
Grated chocolate

Lightly grease a cookie sheet; set aside. Preheat oven to 375°F (190°C). In a medium saucepan, bring butter, corn syrup and brown sugar to a boil, stirring constantly. In a small bowl, combine cocoa, cinnamon, flour and nuts. Gradually stir into hot butter mixture. Drop by level tablespoonfuls about 3 inches apart on prepared cookie sheet. Bake 5 to 6 minutes. Cool about 2 minutes. While still hot, turn cookies over with a spatula, carefully rolling each cookie into a cone shape. If cookies collapse, stuff with small pieces of crumpled aluminum foil until cooled. Place seam-side down on wire rack. If cookies are too firm to roll, return to oven long enough to soften. At serving time, whip cream until it begins to thicken. Add powdered sugar. Continue beating until stiff. Spoon about 2 tablespoons whipped cream into each cone. Sprinkle with grated chocolate. Makes 12 to 14 cones.

How To Make Chantilly Lace Cones

1/These delicate cookies should be removed from the cookie sheets about 2 minutes after coming out of oven. Gently lift each one off with a spatula. Turn cookies over so the rough but more attractive surface will be on the outside.

2/While cookies are still hot, carefully roll into cone shapes. If they collapse, stuff crumpled foil into the centers to hold them until they are set. Cool on metal racks. When cooled, remove the foil. At serving time, fill with whipped cream or ice cream.

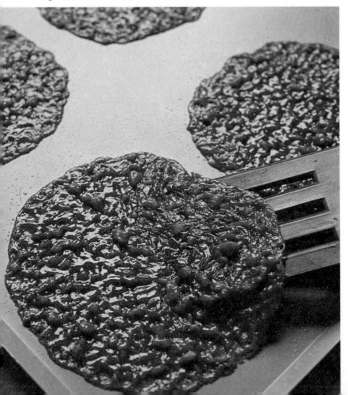

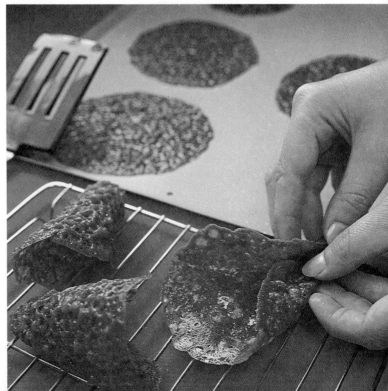

Jumbo Chippers

Make basic cookies or read on for fabulous variations with this basic dough.

1/2 cup butter or margarine	1-1/8 cups flour
1/3 cup granulated sugar	1/2 teaspoon baking soda
1/3 cup light brown sugar, firmly packed	1/2 teaspoon salt
1/2 teaspoon vanilla extract	1 (6-oz.) pkg. semisweet chocolate pieces
1/4 teaspoon water	(1 cup)
1 egg	1/2 cup chopped peanuts

Grease cookie sheets; set aside. Preheat oven to 350°F (175°C). In a large mixer bowl, cream butter or margarine, granulated and brown sugars, vanilla and water. Beat in egg. Add flour, baking soda and salt. Mix well. Stir in chocolate pieces and peanuts. Makes 2-1/2 cups dough. Spread 1/4 cup dough into a 4-inch circle on prepared cookie sheet. Repeat until all dough is used and 10 cookies are formed. Bake 10 to 12 minutes. Place on a wire rack to cool. Makes 10 cookies.

Jumbo Chipper Sandwiches

A child's dream of paradise!

1/4 cup butter or margarine	1/2 teaspoon vanilla extract
1/4 cup peanut butter	3 tablespoons milk
2 cups powdered sugar	10 Jumbo Chippers, cooled, above

In a medium bowl, cream butter or margarine and peanut butter. Add powdered sugar, vanilla and milk. Beat until smooth. Spread generously on 5 Jumbo Chippers. Top with remaining Jumbo Chippers. Makes 5 cookie sandwiches.

Jumbo Chipper Sundaes

Jumbo Chipper dough but make the cookies twice as big!

1 recipe for Jumbo Chipper dough, above	Fudge sauce or chocolate sauce, pages 30 to 40
Vanilla ice cream	Whipped cream
Chocolate ice cream	Chopped peanuts

Grease cookie sheets. Preheat oven to 350° F (175°C). Spread 1/2 cup Jumbo Chipper dough into a 6-inch circle on a prepared cookie sheet. Repeat until all dough is used and 5 cookies are formed. Bake 12 to 15 minutes. Place on a wire rack. When completely cool, place cookies on a serving plate. Put 2 or 3 small scoops of each kind of ice cream on each cookie. Pour fudge or chocolate sauce over ice cream; top with whipped cream and chopped peanuts. Each Jumbo Chipper Sundae makes 2 to 3 servings. If you don't need 5 sundaes, keep the remaining cookies in a covered container and make sundaes when desired. Makes 10 to 15 servings.

For The Calorie-Conscious

What do you miss the most when you're on a diet? Chocolate, of course! Realizing that most calorie-counters are faced with this problem, we have included this chapter of calorie-conscious chocolate recipes. There are no magic potions or unusual ingredients. Just a few popular chocolate recipes where the calories have been reduced. The same basic flavors have been maintained, while some of the rich calorie-laden ingredients have been reduced or substitutes have been used.

For example, non-fat or skim milk is used instead of half-and-half or whipping cream and the amount of butter or margarine is reduced. Although chocolate products used in moderation are not extremely high in calories, we have reduced the amount used in each recipe. As a result, you'll find that these calorie-conscious recipes do not have a strong chocolate flavor. They give the dieter a taste of chocolate without adding many calories. For a more definite chocolate flavor, add an extra square of chocolate or a tablespoon of cocoa.

If you are counting calories but can't resist trying recipes from other sections of this book, consider experimenting on your own. The caloric content in many of the recipes in the previous sections can be lowered by reducing the sugar to 2/3 or less of the amount called for. Keep in mind that the recipes were tested with the specified amounts of sugar and changes in the sugar content may effect the texture of the finished product.

Dieter's Chocolate Pudding

You don't have to give up everything!

2/3 cup sugar
2 tablespoons cornstarch
2 tablespoons unsweetened cocoa powder
1/8 teaspoon salt

2 cups skim milk
2 egg yolks, slightly beaten
1 teaspoon vanilla extract

In a medium saucepan, combine sugar, cornstarch, cocoa and salt. Stir in skim milk and beaten egg yolks. Stir constantly over medium heat until mixture comes to a boil; simmer 1 minute longer. Remove from heat. Stir in vanilla. Pour into a serving bowl. Cover and cool. Makes 5 servings, about 180 calories per serving.

Cinnamon-Chocolate Sauce

A good-tasting, low-calorie topping for angel-food cake or pears.

1 oz. semisweet chocolate, chopped
2 tablespoons sugar
1/4 cup instant nonfat dry milk powder

1/2 cup water
1/4 teaspoon cinnamon

In a small saucepan, combine chopped chocolate, sugar, dry milk powder, water and cinnamon. Stir constantly over low heat until smooth. Makes 1/2 cup sauce, about 35 calories per tablespoon.

Peachy Cocoa Cheesecake

What a treat for dieters!

1/2 cup cornflake crumbs
1 tablespoon sugar
1 tablespoon butter or margarine, melted
1-1/2 cups low-calorie cottage cheese
2 eggs
1/2 cup sugar

1 tablespoon unsweetened cocoa powder
1/2 teaspoon vanilla extract
1/4 teaspoon almond extract
1 (8-oz.) can sliced unsweetened peaches,
   drained

Combine cornflake crumbs with 1 tablespoon sugar and melted butter or margarine. Press into bottom and side of an 8-inch pie pan. Preheat oven to 350°F (175°C). In blender, combine cottage cheese with eggs, 1/2 cup sugar, cocoa, vanilla and almond extract. Blend until almost smooth. Pour into prepared pie pan. Bake 35 to 40 minutes. Refrigerate at least 2 hours. Just before serving, arrange drained peaches on top. Makes 8 servings, about 100 calories per serving.

Angel-Food Strata

Pick up an angel-food cake at the bakery and create a beautiful 3-layer cake.

1/2 cup sugar

1 tablespoon unsweetened cocoa powder

2 tablespoons cornstarch

1-1/4 cups cold water

2 eggs, slightly beaten

1/2 teaspoon vanilla extract

1 (1-lb. 3-oz.) angel-food cake

4 maraschino cherries, halved

In a medium saucepan, combine sugar, cocoa and cornstarch. Stir in water, then eggs. Stir constantly over low heat until thickened and smooth. Remove from heat. Stir in vanilla. Cool until lukewarm. Cut cake horizontally into 3 layers. Spread filling between layers and on top of cake. Garnish with cherries. Makes 10 servings, about 230 calories per serving, to 12 servings, about 180 calories per serving.

How To Make Angel-Food Strata

1/Buy any unfrosted angel food cake at the bakery or make one from a mix. With a sharp serrated knife, cut cake into 3 horizontal slices. Place one slice on a large cake plate.

2/Spread about 1/3 of the slightly cooled chocolate filling between each cake layer. Spread the remaining 1/3 of the filling on top. Decorate with maraschino cherries. Refrigerate until serving time.

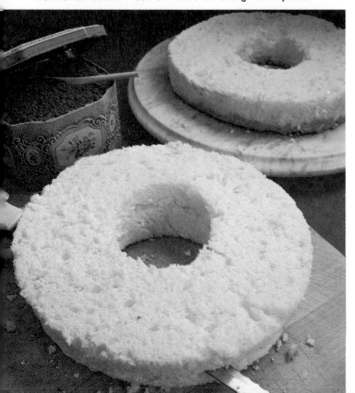

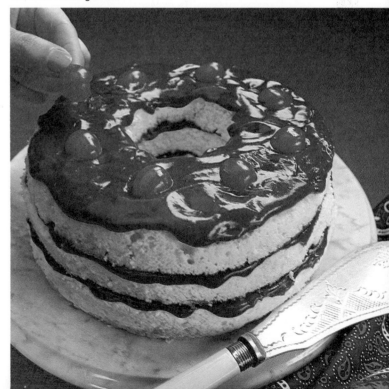

Minted Yogurt Mold

Very smooth and pleasantly tart.

4 ladyfingers
1 envelope unflavored gelatin
2 tablespoons water
1 cup sugar
4 tablespoons unsweetened cocoa powder

1 cup skim milk
1/4 teaspoon peppermint extract
1 cup plain yogurt
2 egg whites
1/8 teaspoon cream of tartar

Halve ladyfingers lengthwise, then halve each crosswise. Stand ladyfinger quarters upright, rounded end up, around side of an 8-inch springform pan; set aside. Sprinkle gelatin over water; set aside to soften. In a medium saucepan, stir together sugar and cocoa. Add skim milk. Bring to a boil over medium-low heat, stirring constantly. Add gelatin mixture. Boil, stirring constantly, over low heat about 10 minutes or until mixture reaches 220°F (105°C) on a candy thermometer. Remove from heat and stir in peppermint extract; set aside to cool 20 to 25 minutes. In a large bowl, stir yogurt until smooth. Blend in cooled chocolate mixture. Refrigerate 20 to 25 minutes. In a small bowl, beat egg whites until foamy. Add cream of tartar. Continue beating until stiff but not dry. Stir a heaping tablespoon of beaten egg whites into chilled chocolate mixture, then fold remaining egg whites into chocolate mixture until blended. Pour into prepared pan. Refrigerate at least 3 hours or overnight. Makes 8 servings, about 160 per serving.

Calorie-Counter's Cake Roll

Chocolate cake rolled up with creamy-crunchy peppermint filling.

5 egg yolks
3/4 cup powdered sugar
1 teaspoon vanilla extract
3 tablespoons unsweetened cocoa powder
5 egg whites

1 envelope low-calorie dessert topping mix
Liquid according to pkg. directions
2 tablespoons crushed peppermint stick candy
Powdered sugar, if desired

Grease a 15" x 10-1/2" pan, line with wax paper and grease wax paper; set aside. Preheat oven to 350°F (175°C). In a small mixer bowl, beat egg yolks until very thick and lemon-colored, about 5 minutes. Gradually add 3/4 cup powdered sugar, beating until mixture is thick again. Mix in vanilla and cocoa. In a large mixer bowl, beat egg whites until stiff but not dry. Carefully fold into egg yolk mixture. Spoon into prepared pan; gently spread until even. Bake 18 to 20 minutes. Sprinkle clean dry dish towel with powdered sugar. As soon as cake is out of oven, loosen sides and turn upside down on prepared dish towel. Remove wax paper. Starting with narrow end, roll up cake and towel together. Cool rolled up cake on wire rack. When cake is cool, whip topping according to package directions. Unroll cake. Spread with whipped topping and sprinkle crushed candy over topping. Reroll cake without towel. If desired, sprinkle with powdered sugar before slicing. Makes 8 servings, about 180 calories per serving.

Lo-Cal Baked Custard

A really good dessert in spite of its few calories.

1/3 cup sugar
1 tablespoon unsweetened cocoa powder
2 eggs, slightly beaten

1/2 teaspoon vanilla extract
1-3/4 cups skim milk
Nutmeg

Preheat oven to 350°F (175°C). In a medium bowl, combine sugar and cocoa. Stir in beaten eggs, vanilla and skim milk. Pour into four 6-ounce custard cups. Sprinkle with nutmeg. Place cups in an 11" x 7" baking pan. Pour almost boiling water into pan around custard cups about 1 inch deep. Bake 45 minutes or until knife inserted into custard comes out clean. Serve warm or cold. Makes 4 servings, about 157 calories per serving.

Snappy Chiffon Pie

Exceptional flavor!

22 chocolate snap cookies
1 envelope unflavored gelatin
1/2 cup skim milk
1 oz. semisweet chocolate, chopped
1/2 cup sugar

1/4 teaspoon salt
2 egg yolks
1 teaspoon vanilla extract
2 egg whites
1/4 cup whipping cream

Place cookies in bottom and around side of an 8-inch pie pan. In a small saucepan, soften gelatin in skim milk. Stir in chopped chocolate, sugar and salt. Stir constantly over low heat until chocolate is completely melted and mixture is smooth. In a medium bowl, beat egg yolks with vanilla. Gradually beat in the hot chocolate mixture. Cool 15 minutes. In a small mixer bowl, beat egg whites until stiff. Fold into chocolate mixture. In a small bowl, whip cream. Fold into chocolate mixture. Spoon into prepared pie pan. Refrigerate several hours. Makes 8 servings, about 180 calories per serving.

Marshmallow Toasties

Graham cracker goodies with a chocolate dot in the center.

8 graham crackers
8 large marshmallows

8 semisweet chocolate pieces

Preheat broiler. Arrange crackers on a cookie sheet. Place a marshmallow on each cracker. Top each marshmallow with a chocolate piece. Broil at least 4 inches from heat until marshmallow tops are toasty brown, about 1 minute. Check frequently to avoid overtoasting. Makes 8 servings, about 56 calories per serving.

Metric Charts

CONVERSION TO METRIC MEASURE

WHEN YOU KNOW	SYMBOL	MULTIPLY BY	TO FIND	SYMBOL
teaspoons	tsp	5	milliliters	ml
tablespoons	tbsp	15	milliliters	ml
fluid ounces	fl oz	30	milliliters	ml
cups	c	0.24	liters	l
pints	pt	0.47	liters	l
quarts	qt	0.95	liters	l
ounces	oz	28	grams	g
pounds	lb	0.45	kilograms	kg
Fahrenheit	°F	5/9 (after subtracting 32)	Celsius	C
inches	in	2.54	centimeters	cm
feet	ft	30.5	centimeters	cm

LIQUID MEASURE TO MILLILITERS

1/4 teaspoon	=	1.25 millileters
1/2 teaspoon	=	2.5 milliliters
3/4 teaspoon	=	3.75 milliliters
1 teaspoon	=	5 milliliters
1-1/4 teaspoons	=	6.25 milliliters
1-1/2 teaspoons	=	7.5 milliliters
1-3/4 teaspoons	=	8.75 milliliters
2 teaspoons	=	10 milliliters
1 tablespoon	=	15 milliliters
2 tablespoons	=	30 milliliters

FAHRENHEIT TO CELSIUS

F	C
200°	93°
225°	107°
250°	121°
275°	135°
300°	149°
325°	163°
350°	177°
375°	191°
400°	205°
425°	218°
450°	232°
475°	246°
500°	260°

LIQUID MEASURE TO LITERS

1/4 cup	=	0.06 liters
1/2 cup	=	0.12 liters
3/4 cup	=	0.18 liters
1 cup	=	0.24 liters
1-1/4 cups	=	0.3 liters
1-1/2 cups	=	0.36 liters
2 cups	=	0.48 liters
2-1/2 cups	=	0.6 liters
3 cups	=	0.72 liters
3-1/2 cups	=	0.84 liters
4 cups	=	0.96 liters
4-1/2 cups	=	1.08 liters
5 cups	=	1.2 liters
5-1/2 cups	=	1.32 liters

Index

9.1385742